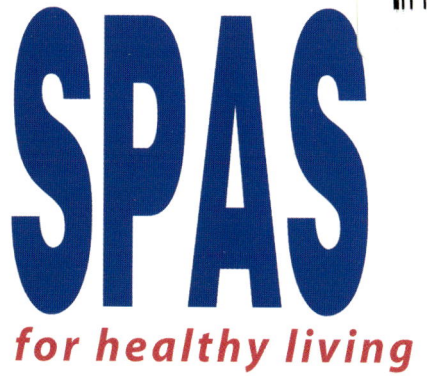

SPAS
for healthy living

Vijaya Kumar

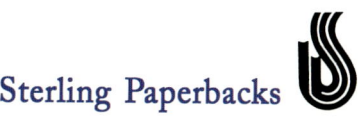
Sterling Paperbacks

STERLING PAPERBACKS
An imprint of
Sterling Publishers (P) Ltd.
A-59, Okhla Industrial Area, Phase-II,
New Delhi-110020.
Tel: 26387070, 26386209; Fax: 91-11-26383788
E-mail: sterlingpublishers@airtelmail.in
ghai@nde.vsnl.net.in
www.sterlingpublishers.com

Spas for Healthy Living
© 2008, Sterling Publishers Pvt. Ltd., New Delhi
ISBN 978 81 207 3891 1

All rights are reserved.
No part of this publication may be reproduced, stored in a retrieval system or transmitted, in any form or by any means, mechanical, photocopying, recording or otherwise, without prior written permission of the original publisher.

Printed and Published by Sterling Publishers Pvt. Ltd., New Delhi-110 020.

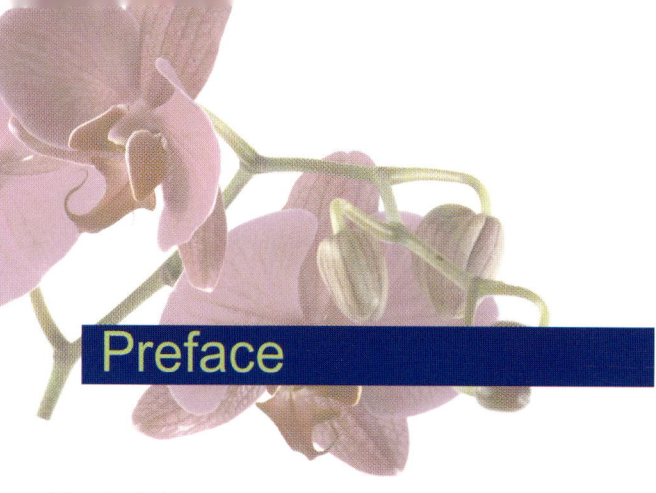

Preface

By definition, a spa is a place where there are curative waters, for instance, thermal or mineral. With this definition, every hotel or resort having a mineral spring can call itself a spa hotel or resort.

The word 'spa' has been taken from the name of famous mineral springs in Spa, Belgium. It has become a common noun denoting any place with a medicinal or mineral spring, or a place where water is believed to have special health-giving properties.

From a very early time, our ancestors enjoyed the benefits of natural hot springs. The evidence of organised use of the thermal spring, dating back 5,000 years, shows that the oldest known spa still in existence is in Merano, Italy. The Egyptians used thermal baths for therapeutic purposes as early as 2000 BC. The Greeks built baths near hot springs and volcanoes around 500 BC. Hippocrates recommended hydrotherapy for the treatment of jaundice and rheumatism. The Romans built elaborate, adequate systems for carrying mineral waters throughout complex private rooms, steam rooms and public baths.

According to the International Spa Association, "Spas are entities devoted to enhancing overall well-being through a variety of professional services that encourage the renewal of mind, body and spirit."

A spa is a good place to go for an extended stay that provides luxurious body treatments. These can include body wraps, baths, massages, manicures, pedicures, body treatments, facials, aromatherapy, nutrition and weight guidance, yoga and meditation.

As we enter the twenty-first century, spa industry promises to be one of the fastest growing segments of the travel industry. More people are becoming aware that the answer to a healthier self is based on a long-term commitment to exercise, a low-fat diet and stress reduction. In that context, spas have become wellness centres that educate people on achieving healthy goals.

This book focuses on the various types of body treatment that you can expect in a spa. Whether you are feeling dull, lethargic or require care for a specific problem, like acne, weight loss, muscle fatigue, stress, or just some general beauty care, a good spa will treat them.

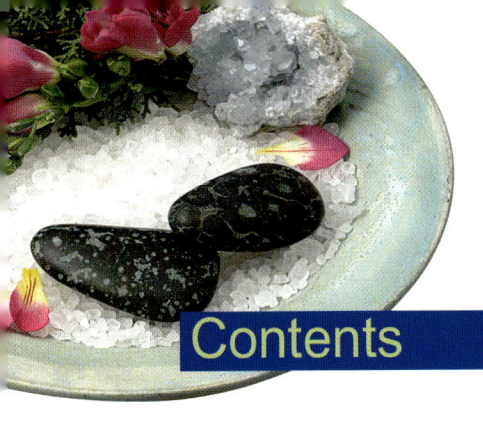

Contents

Preface	3
Kinds of Spas	7
Body Massages	11
Body Scrubs	35
Body Wraps and Polishes	43
Invigorating Baths	50
Beauty Treatments	53
Traditional Indian Spa Treatments	60
Spa Manicure and Pedicure	64
Spa Hair and Other Treatments	71

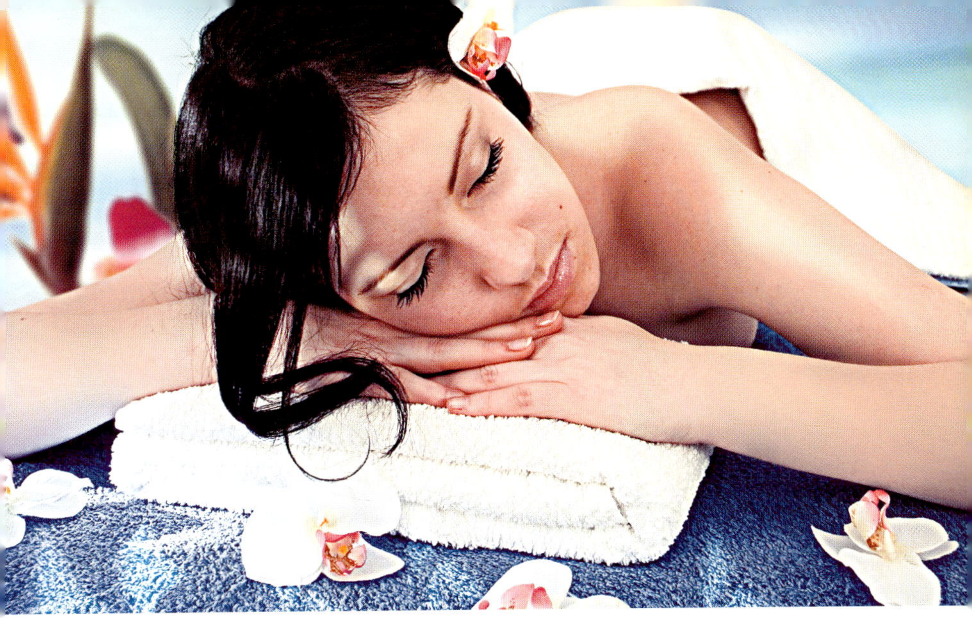

KINDS OF SPAS

A spa has been part of therapeutic healing and health maintenance for ages. Today's spa originated from the ancient custom known as 'taking the waters' in spectacular European health spas.

Spas are wide-ranging from world-class getaway destination spas to superior day spas in vibrant city locations. All provide rejuvenating, relaxing and luxurious spa treatments.

There are many types of spas, though the main ones are the day spa, the destination spa and the resort spa. More recently, the medical spa has been popping up.

Day Spa

A day spa, the most common kind of spa, is usually a clean, safe and nurturing environment offering a menu of spa treatments administered by highly trained professionals. This is for people who want to drop in for one or two treatments, or perhaps even indulge in a half day session.

Day spas are getting away from long, confusing menus, and focusing on treatments such as massage, facials, body treatments and other mainstays on a day-use basis. Most offer manicures and pedicures as well.

Facilities will vary at day spas, but most have treatment rooms, a waiting room and a tiled room with special shower facilities for more elaborate treatments.

Destination Spa

A destination spa is a place where you can participate in a variety of exclusively structured programmes, including weight loss, nutrition, a fitness regime, healing, meditation and yoga. A total renewal of the mind, body and spirit is offered at the destination spa.

The destination spa gives a complete spa experience in an overnight setting (most require a two- or three-night minimum stay). Its sole purpose is to provide mind and body fitness, healthy eating, spa treatments and relaxation.

The facilities of the destination spas are more elaborate and extensive than the average day spas. Ideally, it will have hydrotherapy tubs, wet rooms, steam baths and saunas, jacuzzis, and some unusual treatments. You can expect a wide selection of exercise and stress-reduction classes, as well as outdoor

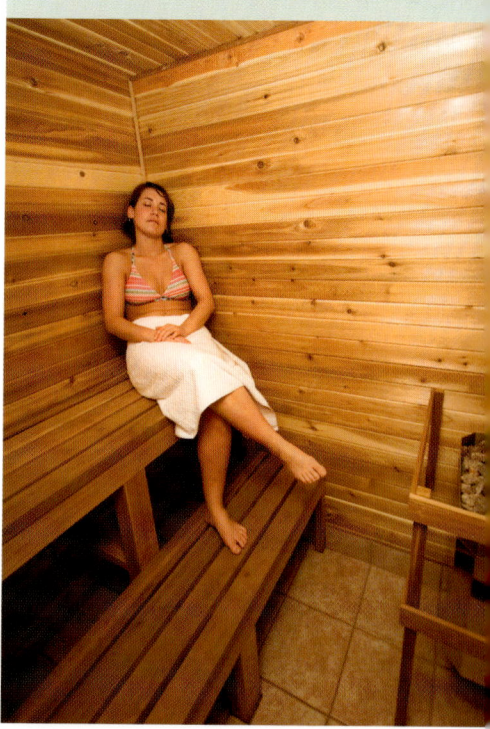

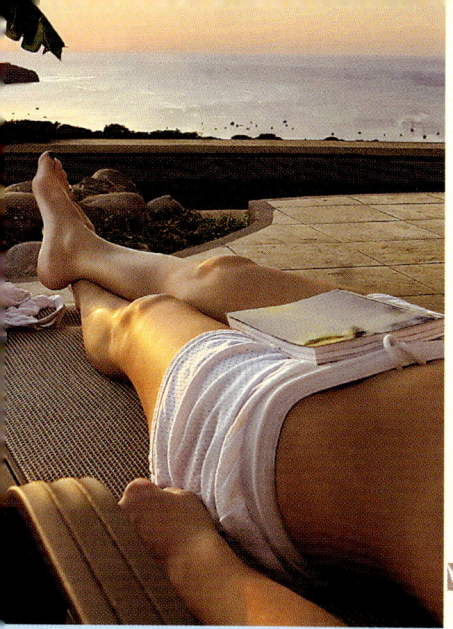

activities. It has gyms for working out, swimming pools, tennis courts, and a meditation centre.

At destination spas, the whole environment is geared towards fitness, healthy eating, relaxation and experience. Prices generally include all meals and regular exercise classes. Spa treatments like massage, facials and body treatments are sometimes included in the package, but often they are extra.

Resort Spa

Resort spas come in a wide range of sizes and styles.

Resort or hotel spas are often located close to a natural spring source. Here guests who enjoy the spa concept can take advantage of traditional resort activities. They can combine vacations along with the amenities the modern spa has to offer.

Resort spas continue to diversify their treatment offerings with indigenous experiences, like Thai massage, Ashtanga, Indian head massage, Ayurveda, Shiatsu and hot stone massage which are popular treatments.

Medical Spa

Medical spas, also known as medi spas, blend traditional medical expertise with spa luxury and innovation. Medical spas are becoming trusted venues for executives, physicals, health and wellness programmes, cosmetic treatments, dentistry and dermatology.

Eco Spa

Eco spas are environment-friendly destinations. They believe that personal health begins with global health – a belief that extends to the way they create spa products (all organic ingredients), wash dishes (vinegar instead of soap), light rooms (solar panels and fluorescent bulbs) and process waste water (bacteria, fish, snails, etc.). In short, eco spas offer all the luxuries of a traditional spa but use of chemical and processed elements are strictly limited, the emphasis being on natural elements.

Ayurvedic Spa

This type of spa is based on the ancient Indian practice of traditional folk medicine. It includes nutrition, herbal therapy, aromatherapy, massage and meditation.

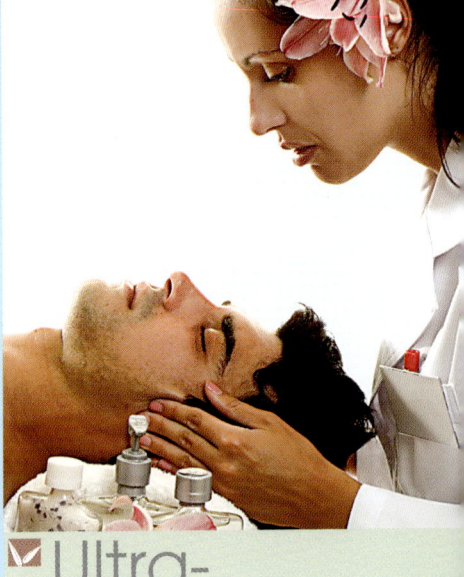

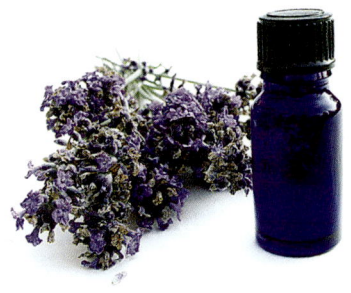

Men-only Spa

A growing number of men are going to spas these days. And they are not just signing up for sports massages and manicure, they are bellying up for cocoa butter rub downs and seaweed body wraps.

Ultra-luxurious Spas

The luxury end of the market is becoming even more luxurious. That trend is in two directions: at one end you have a more exclusive, tasteful experience, such as the Mandarin Oriental's Asian-inspired spas; on the other hand, you have the 'bling' factor, like creams made with diamonds. Stay tuned for daily private spiritual and wellness counselling, ruby/diamond/emerald/sapphire massage oils, four-hour massages, three-therapist treatments, underwater spas, private hotel/spa rooms, and a slate of ultra-chic big-name designer spas.

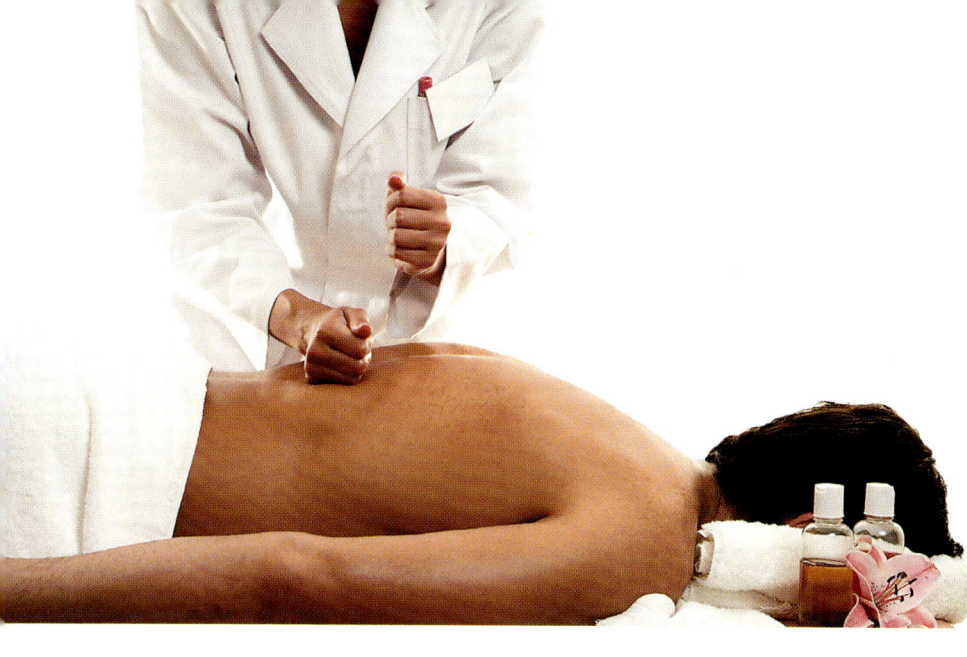

BODY
MASSAGES

A massage is the practice of applying pressure or vibration to the soft tissues of the body, including muscles, connective tissues, tendons, ligaments and joints. Massage can be applied to parts of the body, or successively to the whole body, to heal injury, relieve psychological stress, manage pain, improve blood circulation, and relieve tension.

A massage therapist assesses clients by conducting a range of motion and muscle testing, and proposes suitable treatment plans. All health resorts provide good body massage treatments, offering you various packages and options.

SPAS

History of Massage

Massage is the oldest and simplest form of medical care and therapy. This can be corroborated by ancient Egyptian tomb paintings depicting people being massaged. In Eastern cultures, massage is being practised continually since ancient times. *The Yellow Emperor's Classic of Internal Medicine,* a Chinese book from 2700 BC, recommends "breathing exercises, massage of skin and flesh, and exercises of hands and feet" as the appropriate treatment for "complete paralysis, chills and fever". Massage was one of the principal methods of relieving pain for Greek and Roman physicians.

Ayurveda, the traditional Indian system of medicine, places great emphasis on the therapeutic benefits of massage with aromatic oils and spices. It is practised very widely in India, especially in the state of Kerala.

Swedish massage, the method most familiar to Westerners, was reported to be developed in the nineteenth century.

Physiotherapy was established with the foundation in 1894 of the Society of Trained Masseurs in Europe.

However, later breakthroughs in medical technology and pharmacology eclipsed massage, as physiotherapists began favouring electrical instruments over manual methods of stimulating the tissues.

Massage Therapy

Today, massage is considered to be a holistic therapy.

Therapeutic massage complements medical treatment by making people feel less stressed and anxious, relaxed and yet more alert.

Massage is now used in intensive care units for children, elderly people, babies in incubators, and patients with cancer, AIDS, heart attacks or strokes.

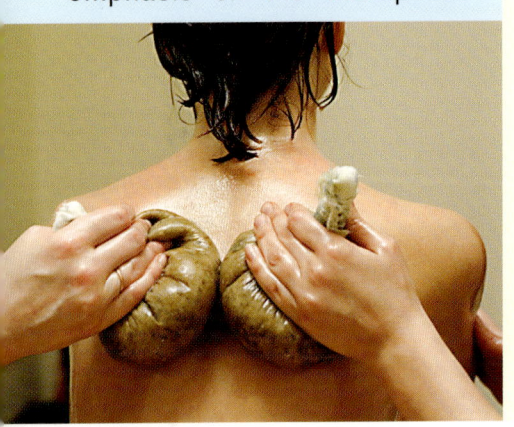

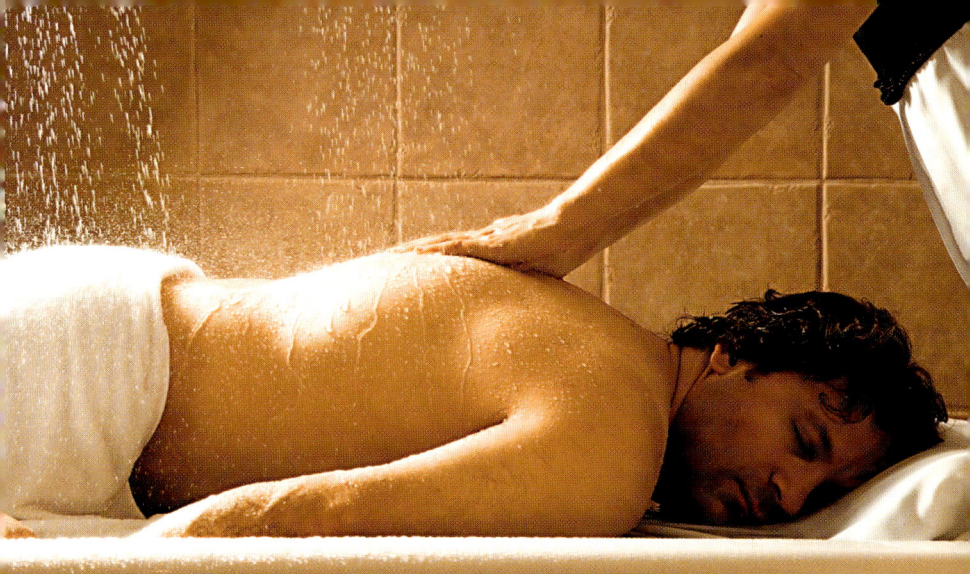

A variety of massage techniques have also been incorporated into several other complementary therapies, such as reflexology, aromatherapy, osteopathy, rolfing and hellerwork.

Benefits of Massage

1. Massage has an effect on both body and mind. It also has a beneficial effect on the internal organs and the immune system.

2. It increases the circulation of blood and flow of lymph. Lymph is a milky white fluid that drains impurities and wastes away from the tissue cells.

3. Massage reduces muscle tension. It loosens contracted, shortened, hardened muscles. It can stimulate and strengthen weak, flaccid muscles.

4. The oxygen capacity of the blood can increase 10 to 15 per cent after a massage, and relieves chronic pain.

5. Massage enhances the condition of the skin by improving the function of the sebaceous and sweat glands that keep the skin clean, lubricated and cool.

6. Massage results in better digestion and intestinal function.

7. Massage alleviates discomfort during pregnancy.

8. It reduces blood pressure, and relieves one of tension-related headaches and eye-strains.

Types of Massages

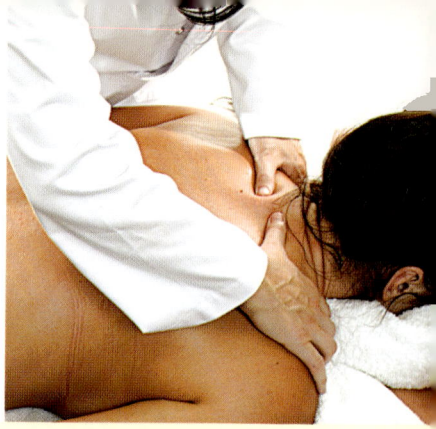

All health resorts offer a variety of massages that prove beneficial, both physically and mentally. Generally, they all offer the following:
1. Swedish massage
2. Chinese massage
3. Thai massage
4. Shiatsu massage
5. Hawaiian (Lomilomi) massage
6. Balinese massage

Swedish Massage

The Swedish massage is a classic full-body massage employing long, kneading strokes that help to promote total relaxation and ease muscle stress.

History

Swedish massage did not originate in Sweden. There is no Swedish massage in Sweden. Instead, the massage is referred to almost universally as 'classic massage'.

Swedish massage, or classic massage, is generally credited to the Dutch practitioner, Johan Georg Mezger (1838-1909), and endorsed by physicians, such as Emil Kleen and Richard Hael who researched the origins of massage and gymnastics. Mezger adopted the French terms – *effleurage, petrissage* and *tapotement* to denote the basic strokes under which he systematised massage as we know it today.

Basic Techniques of Swedish Massage

Swedish massage currently represents the Western standard for massage. Also known as 'therapeutic massage', it represents a general massage system that focuses on increasing circulation and promoting relaxation.

The Swedish approach classifies five types of strokes: Effleurage (gliding), Petrissage (kneading), Tapotement (pounding), Friction (rubbing) and Vibration (shaking).

Effleurage

This basic technique of Swedish massage consists of long gliding strokes from the neck down to the base of the spine, or from the shoulder down to the fingertips. When done on the limbs, all strokes are toward the heart to aid blood and lymphatic flow. It is done with the whole hand, or the thumb pads.

involves the motions of kneading and compression, i.e., rolling, squeezing or pressing the muscles to enhance deeper circulation. Petrissage attempts to increase circulation with clearing out toxins from muscle and nerve tissues.

Tapotement

In this technique, using a series of briskly applied percussive movements, the hands are used alternately to strike or tap the muscles for an invigorating effect. This stroke has many variations. It can be applied with the edge of the hand, with the tips of fingers, or with a closed fist. Tapotement attempts to release tension and cramping from muscles in spasms.

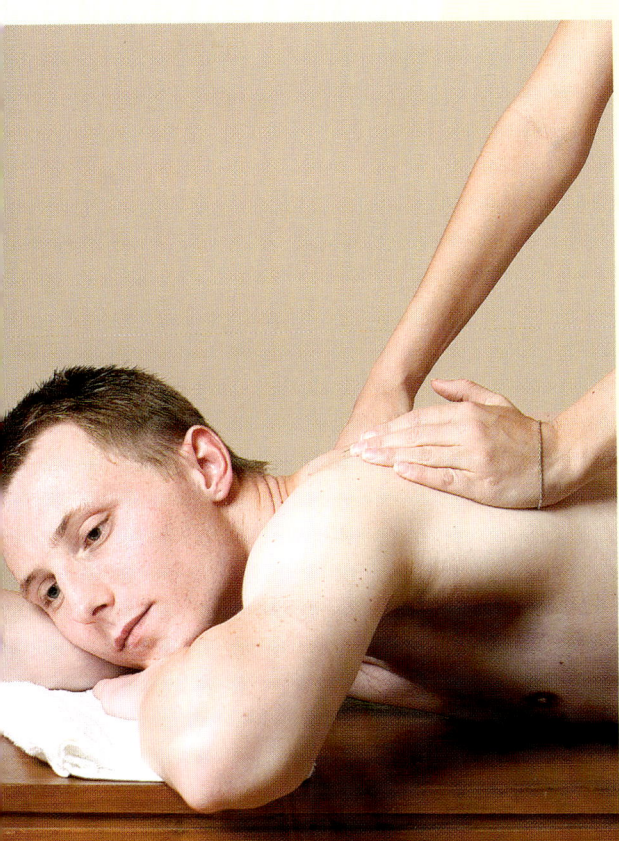

Petrissage

This involves gently lifting muscles up and away from the bones, then rolling and squeezing them, again with a gentle pressure. Basically, it

Friction

This is the most penetrating of the strokes, and consists of deep, circular or transverse movements made with the thumb pads or fingertips. The therapist applies deep, circular

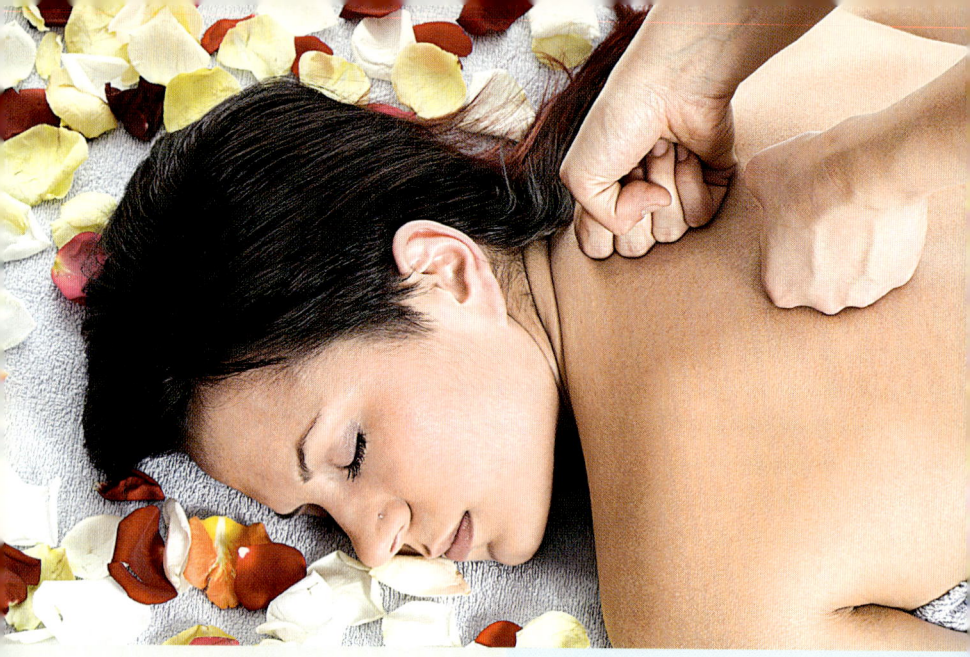

movement near joints and other bony areas (such as the sides of the spine). Friction breaks down adhesions, which are knots resulting when muscle fibres bind together during the healing process, thus contributing to more flexible muscles and joints.

Vibration

For this, the therapist presses his or her hands on the back or limbs, and rapidly shakes the area for a few seconds. This boosts circulation, and increases the power of the muscles to contract or stretch. Vibration is particularly helpful to people suffering from low back pain.

Swedish massage is the foundation for other types of Western massage, including sports, deep tissue and aromatherapy. It is a genre that includes the intentional and systematic manipulation of the soft tissues of the body to enhance health and healing. Joint movements and stretching are commonly performed as part of the massage. Since the strokes are light and rhythmic, Swedish massages are enjoyed by people of all ages and lifestyles.

Chinese Massage

If you are unwell or in pain then Chinese massage, known as *Tui Na,* can give you welcome relief. It is simply the most tried and tested massage therapy in the world. It is a very effective treatment when used in combination with acupuncture. The Chinese massage combines stretching, long strokes, skin rolling, and palm and thumb pressure techniques that promote relaxation and a sense of harmony.

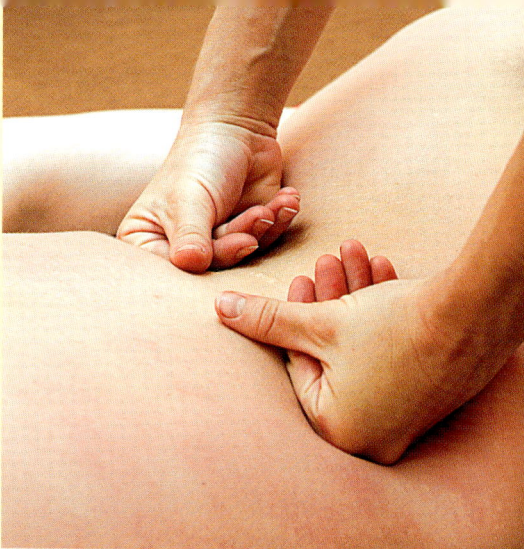

History

Chinese massage is a form of manual medicine dating back almost three thousand years. Tui Na (pronounced 'tweenah') massage, acupuncture and Chinese herbal medicine are the three main components of Traditional Chinese Medicine (TCM).

The Chinese adapted massage into work fitness programmes, fighting martial arts, and mainstream medicine. Chinese folk medicine was based in Chinese Tui Na massage for hundreds of years.

Basic Techniques of Chinese Massage

Several concepts are important in understanding the major forms of Chinese massage:
a) Qi
b) Jing luo
c) Xue
d) Jin

Qi: Sometimes spelt as *chi* or *ki,* Qi is the basic life energy animating the universe as well as human beings. The word can be translated into English as 'breath' or 'air'. Qi can be transferred or transmuted. In humans, the digestive tract extracts the qi from food, while the lungs extract it from air. When these two forms of qi meet in the bloodstream, they form human qi, which then circulates throughout the body.

Jing luo: The meridians or channels known as jing luo are a network of energy pathways that link and balance the various organs. When these meridians are blocked, the qi and blood cannot circulate smoothly, and the person experiences physical pain.

Xue: They are acupoints or locations on the body where qi tends to collect, and can be manipulated or redirected. They are connected to different body organs through the meridians.

Jin: The soft and connective tissues, known as jin, and the joints all affect the flow of qi along the meridians. Thus one function of Chinese massage is to relax the client's jin.

Chinese massage is sometimes described as a combination of several traditional techniques, such as:
1. Tui Na (push and pull)
2. Anmo (rub and press)
3. Dian xue (acupoints)
4. Wai Qi Liao Fa (energy work)
5. Hybrid Chinese massage

The hybrid Chinese massage is a carefully formulated combination of techniques integrated into a 60 or 90 minute session.

Tui Na

Tui Na is an oriental bodywork therapy that has been used in China for 2,000 years. It is a more sophisticated form of manual bodywork than Swedish massage.

Tui Na *(tui* meaning 'push' and *na* meaning 'grasp') was officially incorporated into Traditional Chinese Medicine (TCM) as a medical therapy to be used for problems where acupuncture and herbs were less effective.

Tui Na, one of the earliest medical forms, can be seen in the medical history of every ancient nation in the world. The ancient Chinese folk used to rub, press, knead, pound or stamp on themselves or their fellow bodies in order to keep out cold, get rid of discomfort, and treat various injuries; continually developing their practical experiences, which gradually became what is now known as a natural therapy.

Tui Na is a medical method in which arms, fingers, elbows, hands and knees are used as tools for treating diseases and illnesses. It addresses specific injuries, fitness needs and health conditions through a variety of specialised manipulation techniques.

Tui Na works with the energy system in the body known as the meridian system. Like acupuncture,

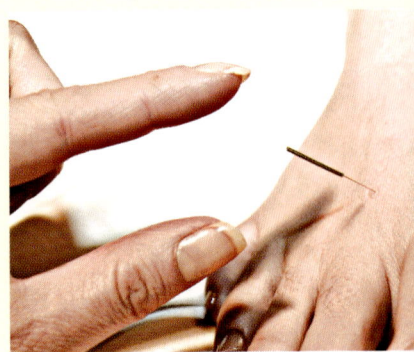

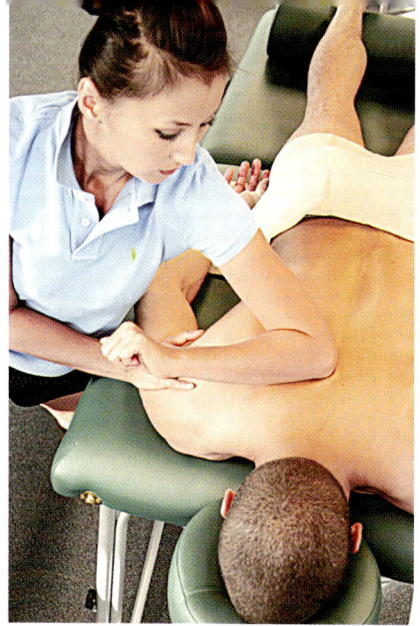

Tui Na works with the qi energy of the patient to bring a balanced state of health. But unlike acupuncture, no needles are used. The work is done entirely with the practitioner's hands to help increase the beneficial flow of qi through the patient's meridian system.

Tui Na treatments are usually applied on top of loose clothing, rarely on the skin directly, although herbal rubs can be used in conjunction with a Tui Na treatment. Some therapists use external herbal poultices, compresses, liniments and salves to enhance the other therapeutic methods, and to facilitate quicker healing. Each session of this massage may last for 30 minutes to one hour.

Tui Na massage is beneficial in many ways:

1. It is well suited for treatment of specific musculo-skeletal disorders and chronic stress-related disorders of the digestive, respiratory and reproductive systems.

2. Tui Na massage treats chronic pain. Neck, shoulder and back pain, immobility, sciatica and tennis elbow, all respond very well.

3. Headaches, migraines, constipation and a whole range of emotional problems improve with a Tui Na therapy by improving the overall qi status of the body.

4. For soft tissue injuries, Tui Na relaxes muscles and tendons, and promotes smooth passage of the channels.

5. It restores natural self-healing abilities and promotes blood circulation. It also removes blood clots.

6. Tui Na may be applied to treat many disorders from soft tissue injuries to many other kinds of ailments such as rheumatic pain, tiredness, lack of energy and any symptom caused by stress or emotional problems.

7. Tui Na is even used for cosmetic purposes such as weight loss and an alternative to botox.

8. It regulates the nervous system and strengthens the body's resistance to disease.

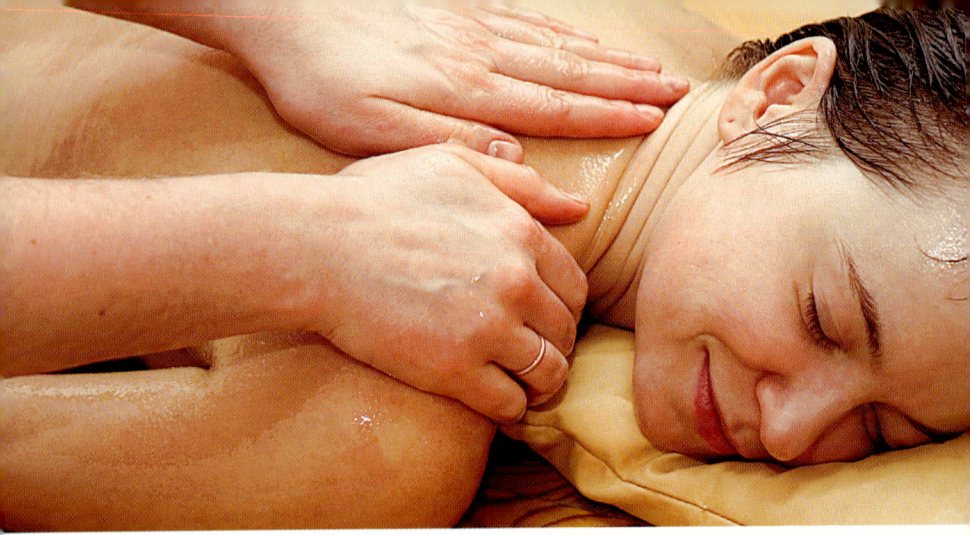

Anmo Massage

Anmo is a type of massage used for health maintenance and to restore vitality. Its name means 'press and stroke' in Chinese. It can be used at home but is also a part of martial arts, qigong and athletic training.

Anmo differs from Tui Na massage in ways that it is a full-body balanced treatment. It combines yang techniques to break up stagnant and sluggish qi and activate its flow, followed by yin techniques to soothe and calm the body.

Anmo is the most common form of Chinese massage. It is an excellent treatment for sore muscles, overworked bodies, athletic and flexibility needs. It has a set pattern of movements and techniques that the therapist follows, but these can be adjusted to the client's needs.

Dian Xue Massage

Dian xue, or 'point press', is familiar to many as acupressure. This is a

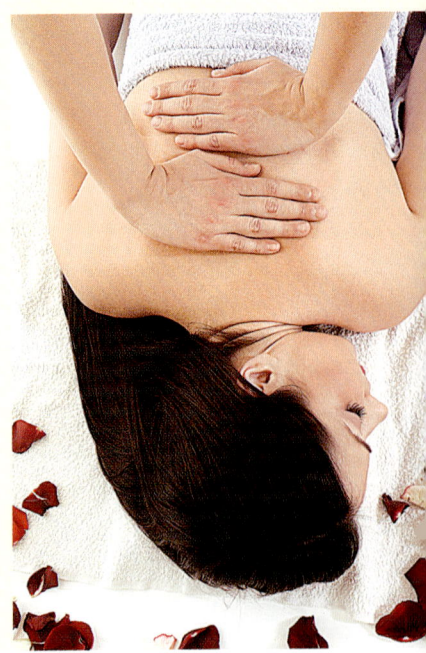

massage without needles that is associated with acupuncture. Dian xue uses the same acupoints and meridians on the body as acupuncture, but relies on pressure from the fingers rather than needles.

Dian xue can be used by masseurs to stimulate two different acupoints, one with each hand, while the area of the body between the points is stretched or twisted to maximise the flow of qi.

Wai Qi Liao Fa

This is a curative healing technique based on the idea that a healer's energy can be used to influence the energy of the patient, perhaps to push or otherwise shift the patient's own energy into a more balanced state, as a means of supporting the natural self-healing process. The Chinese name of this form of massage means 'curing with external qi'. In qi healing, a masseur who has practised the art for many years transmits qi directly to the patient.

Hybrid Chinese Massage

People who require or request for a deeper manual manipulation of muscles and soft tissues get a hybrid combination of different Chinese massage techniques. The

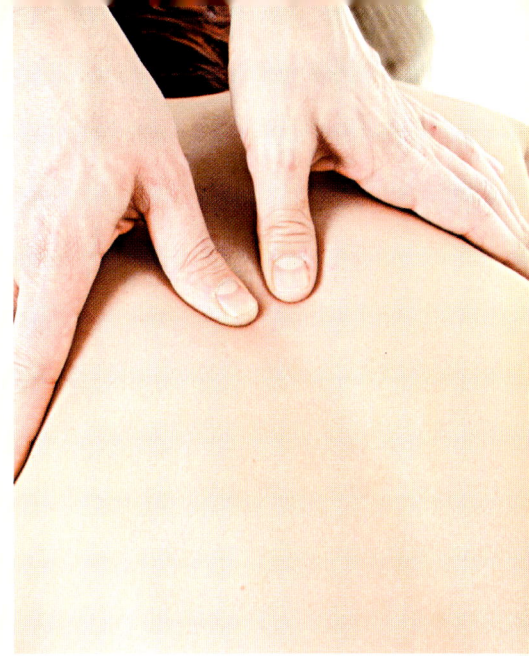

hybrid massage may include grasping and kneading methods combined with stronger soft tissue manipulations typically known as 'deep tissue massage'. It also incorporates flushing and energy balancing methods from acupressure and traditional healing massage methods which prove beneficial especially to athletes, serious trainees and other sports people.

Thai Massage

Thai massage is a unique and wonderful form of hands-on healing work. It can provide a good opportunity of achieving a state of deep mental and emotional equanimity, profound stress relief and moments of sweet bliss.

History

Thai massage was believed to have been developed by Jivaka Kumar Bhaccha, physician to Buddha, more than 2,500 years ago in India. From there, it was brought to Thailand where the techniques and principles gradually became influenced by the Chinese healing system and acupressure techniques.

Basic Techniques of Thai Massage

Traditional Thai massage is based on an energetic paradigm of the human body/mind.

The techniques of Thai massage are applied very slowly. The slowness of practice facilitates the tendency towards mindfulness. Additionally, because many of the techniques require heightened flexibility of the practitioner and the recipient, the slowness significantly diminishes the chances for injury.

Thai massage is usually performed with the recipient wearing loose fitting clothing while lying on a cotton mat on the floor. No oils or lotions are utilised in Thai massage, and the session usually lasts a minimum of 90 minutes.

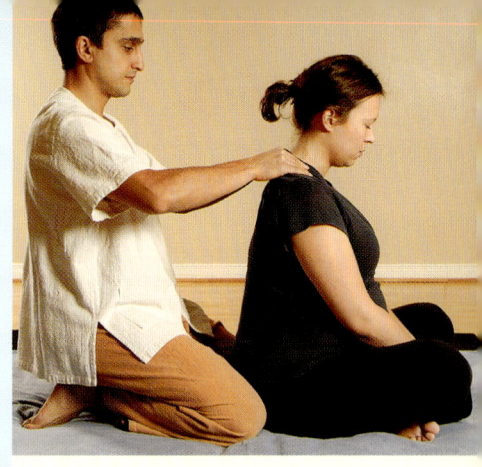

Thai Foot Massage

Thai foot massage is a massage of the lower legs and feet. It involves stretching to open 'Sen' (energy) lines, along with the use of a stick to stimulate the reflex points on the feet which correspond to the internal organs of the body. This massage stimulates these points to promote general health and well-being.

A treatment in Thai foot massage will usually last for an hour, and the therapist may spend the last ten minutes massaging the hands, and sometimes the shoulders too.

Traditional Thai massage and Thai foot massage complement each other beautifully. Thai massage balances the elements of the mind and body, while Thai foot massage stimulates the internal organs, giving the receiver a holistic treatment.

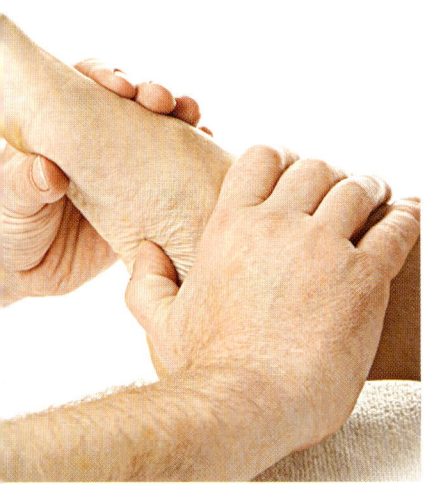

The benefits of a Thai foot massage are:
1. Improved circulation and toxin removal.
2. Stimulated lymphatic drainage and immune system boost.
3. Reduced stiffness and improved flexibility.
4. Accelerated physical healing.
5. Stress relief.
6. Improved sleep and clarity of mind.

Shiatsu Massage

Shiatsu is a form of Japanese massage based on acupressure, and the same principles as acupuncture. Designed to release tension and improve circulation and vital organ function, this method has been practised for centuries in Japan. The treatment involves the rhythmic application of pressure in varying degrees throughout the body to balance energy flow and direct stimulation through certain pathways of the body.

History

Shiatsu is a Japanese healing system that allows the patient or client to get in touch with his or her own healing abilities. It is deeply rooted in the philosophy and practices of traditional Chinese medicine, incorporating the therapeutic massage of Japan, and more recently embracing its original focus of meditation and self-healing.

Shiatsu comes from 'anmo', meaning 'massage'. It was recommended for people living in

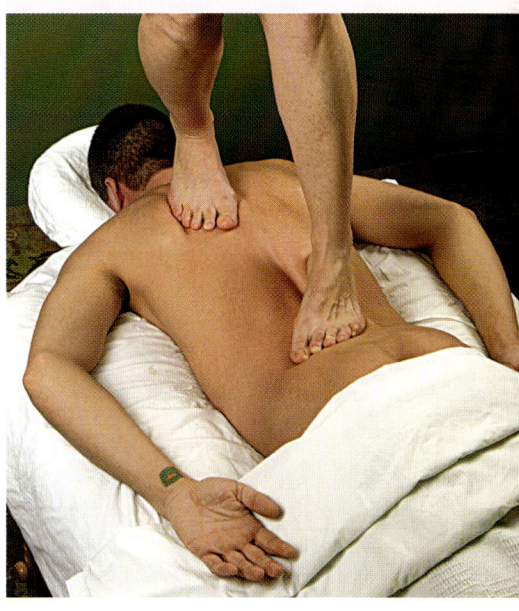

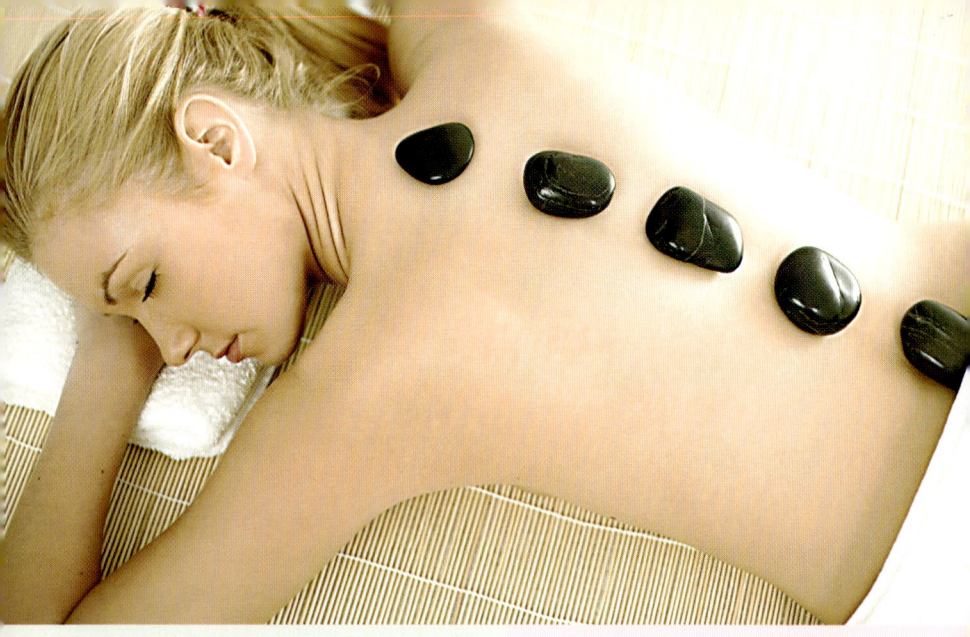

the heart of the country near the Yellow river, where the culture was most developed, and people were doing more mental than physical work. The Japanese borrowed many beneficial techniques from the Chinese culture — anmo and acupuncture — and thus developed it into 'Shiatsu'.

Basically, five types of treatment were practised: acupuncture, medicines and herbs, stone therapy, moxa and anmo.

Basic Techniques of Shiatsu Massage

Usually Shiatsu is defined as an Oriental massage, but it is much more than that. It acts through pressure with thumbs, fingers and palms applied to determined areas and points of the human body, without the use of any mechanical instrument, correcting internal dysfunctions, promoting and keeping the health and treating specific illnesses.

Shiatsu literally means *finger pressure*. Natural body weight is used when pressure is applied on special points on the body.

Shiatsu can be done with the patient lying on a mat on the floor, or on a table. The patient remains fully clothed, i.e., wearing loose-fitting clothing. The atmosphere in the area should be calm and soothing with soft lighting and light music playing in the background. The practitioner's hands are placed at various points of the body, sending the energies to more than

300 acupoints along the way, thus creating the healing.

Shiatsu is a combination of many different techniques, including pressing, hooking, gliding, shaking, rotating, grasping, patting, vibrating, plucking, lifting, pinching, rolling, brushing, and in some spas, walking on the person's legs, feet and back. Therapists apply pressure using their thumbs, palms, elbows and even knees, as well as fingertips. A treatment session will also include gentle stretching of the limbs.

Benefits

1. Shiatsu massage treats common psychological and physical problems by pressing pressure points. It alleviates disorders such as depression, anxiety, nausea, stiffness, headaches, arthritis, cramps or pulled muscles.
2. It reduces stress and fatigue accumulated in the body.
3. It increases circulation of blood and lymph.

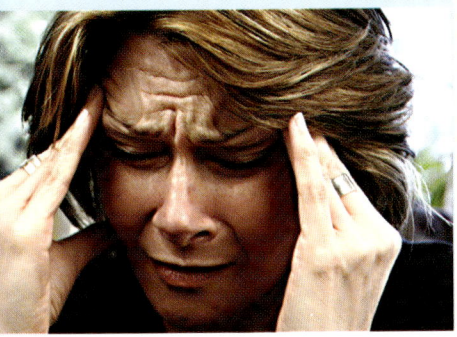

4. It increases vitality, stamina and energy.
5. It stimulates the circulation and flow of lymphatic fluid. It releases toxins, and deep-seated tensions from the muscles.
6. It stimulates the nervous system and the immune system.
7. It improves the functioning of the digestive system.
8. It improves the endocrine system and fortifies the functioning of the organs.

Hawaiian Lomilomi Massage

Lomilomi is a massage therapy that has been practised by the Hawaiians for many centuries. Much more than simply a physical technique, Lomilomi involves a holistic approach to the person, and seeks to heal and promote wellness in body, mind and spirit.

History

Lomilomi, meaning 'massage' in Hawaiian, is an ancient therapy from the Hawaiian healing specialists. They were taught their art for over 20 years, and received their last instructions from their master on his deathbed.

Lomilomi is one of the most profound forms of massage. It is a unique healing massage derived from the ancient Polynesians, and more specifically the master healers of Hawaii.

Basic Techniques of Lomilomi Massage

A Lomilomi usually commences with a stillness between the practitioner and the client, often with the practitioner's hands resting gently on the client's back. The massage is given in fluid, rhythmic motion, using the forearms as well as the hands. Some people have described this feeling as gentle waves moving over their body. Another feature is that different parts of the body may be massaged at the same time; for example, one arm or hand may be working on a shoulder, and the other hand may be working on the opposite hip.

Full body strokes also help to free the energy, make the body soft, promoting free and abundant flow of energy in the recipient. According to Huna philosophy, energy also gets blocked in the joints. Gentle stretches of the body, and gentle rotations of the joints are therefore also incorporated to assist the release of tensions, and assist the flow of energy, once again, not forcefully but feeling the level of the client's resistance or comfort.

The Hawaiians look at things in terms of energy flow, following the idea that a belief can block energy flow as much as muscle tension can. Lomilomi helps release the blockages, whilst at the same time giving the energy a new direction. It also relieves stress and tension, improves blood and lymph flow, eliminates wastes and toxins from the system. Thus Lomilomi not only heals a person physically but also mentally, emotionally and spiritually.

Balinese Massage

This relaxing massage has been handed down through generations. It originated in the Spice Islands of Indonesia.

This massage helps to clear energy and meridian lines using deep compression and deep muscular moves. Partly given dry, then a warming combination of coconut and ginger oils are used to massage deeper into the muscle.

Spas in Bali are devoted to pampering both mind and body. Beautiful sacred spaces, delivering one or the client to a place of peace, serenity and contentment, where aroma, colour and sound blend together to relax, replenish and enliven the spirit.

Balinese spa treatments are a gentle seduction of the body, mind and spirit. It helps in healing, nurturing and relaxing weary souls that are worn out from the demands of everyday living.

The techniques used in Balinese massage include percussion, long and firm strokes, stretching, acupressure (especially on the feet), and the use of aromatic oils such as ylang-ylang, sandalwood, jasmine and vetiver.

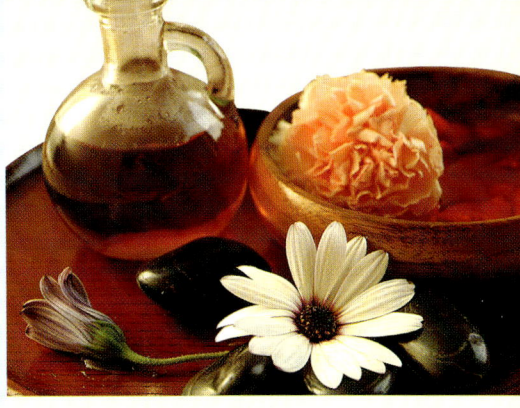

The Balinese massage session lasts for an hour. It uses the techniques of skin rolling, long kneading strokes, foot massage and acupressure which are believed to renew, strengthen and heal the body. Combined with body scrub, baths and wraps, Balinese massage is truly tempting in spas.

Other Types of Massages

Sports Massage

Massage has become an integral part of the new athletic regime from sports medicine clinic to college training rooms to Olympic training. A growing number of trainers believe that massage can provide an extra edge to the sportspersons who participate in high performance sports.

Each sport and athletic event uses muscle groups in a different way. Sports massage therapists

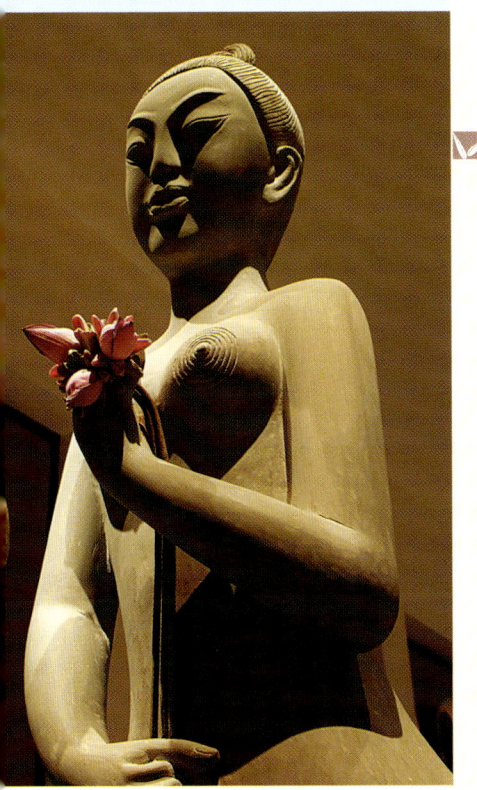

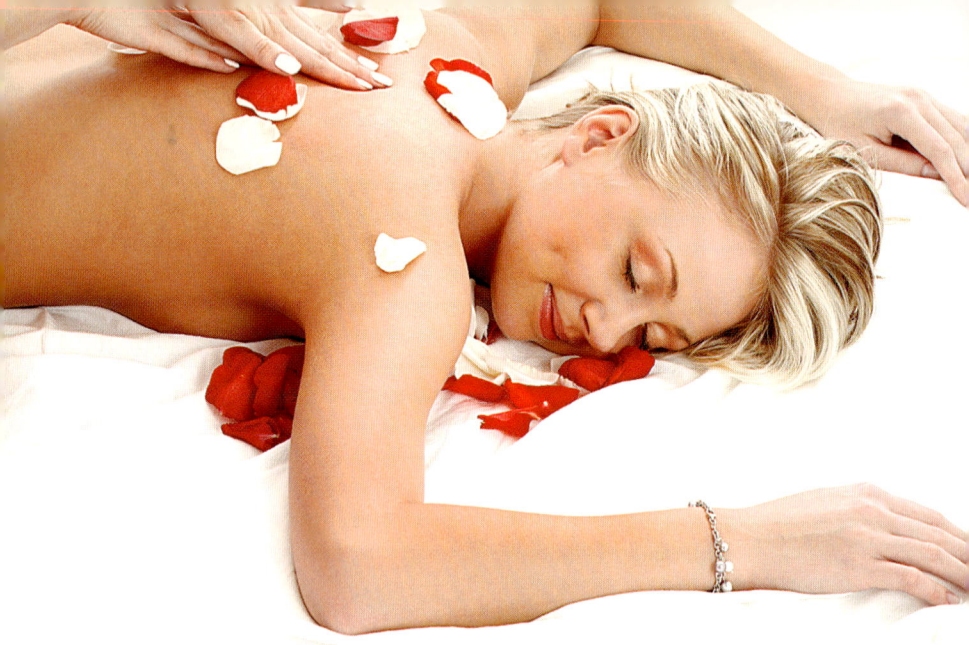

must be familiar with each muscle, the muscle groups and how they are affected by the specific movements and stresses of each sport. They are also trained in the appropriate uses of hydrotherapy and cryotherapy.

Therapeutic massage helps the body recover from the stresses of strenuous exercises, and facilitates the rebuilding phase of conditioning. In addition to general recovery, massage may also focus on specific muscles used in a sport or fitness activity.

Regular sports massage can reduce the chance of injury through proper stretching and event preparation, and also through deep tissue massage.

Sports massage may involve prevention and maintenance programmes, on-site treatment before and after a sports event, and rehabilitation programmes for those who are injured during the programme.

Aromatherapy Massage

Aromatherapy massage awakens your senses with its powerful effects, using a combination of essential oils and Swedish massage techniques. This helps to alleviate your day-to-day stress, and to relax, energise and detoxify. Aromatherapy massage also helps in increasing blood circulation, and in soothing the body, mind and spirit.

Aromatherapy also offers a variation in the form of Raindrop Aromatherapy Massage which is a powerful healing treatment, incorporating four modalities: Swedish massage, reflexology, aromatherapy and energy work. It focuses on the spine, and is designed to release blockages and align energy throughout the body. The essential oils offered in most spas include sandalwood oil, ylang-ylang and spice oils, lavender, lemongrass and nutmeg.

The light, rhythmic strokes with movements toward the lymphatic areas produce gentle relaxation. The deep strokes and cross-fibre massage techniques stimulate the overall blood circulation, while relieving stress, muscle tension and aches in problem areas, especially chronic back pain.

Deep Tissue Massage

Deep tissue massage interacts the most with the body's muscles and muscle groups.

It consists of slower strokes and more pressure. The therapist targets muscle groups after warming the soft tissues. This massage is used to help break up scar tissue.

Trigger Point Therapy Massage

Trigger points are tender areas usually found in tight muscles. They

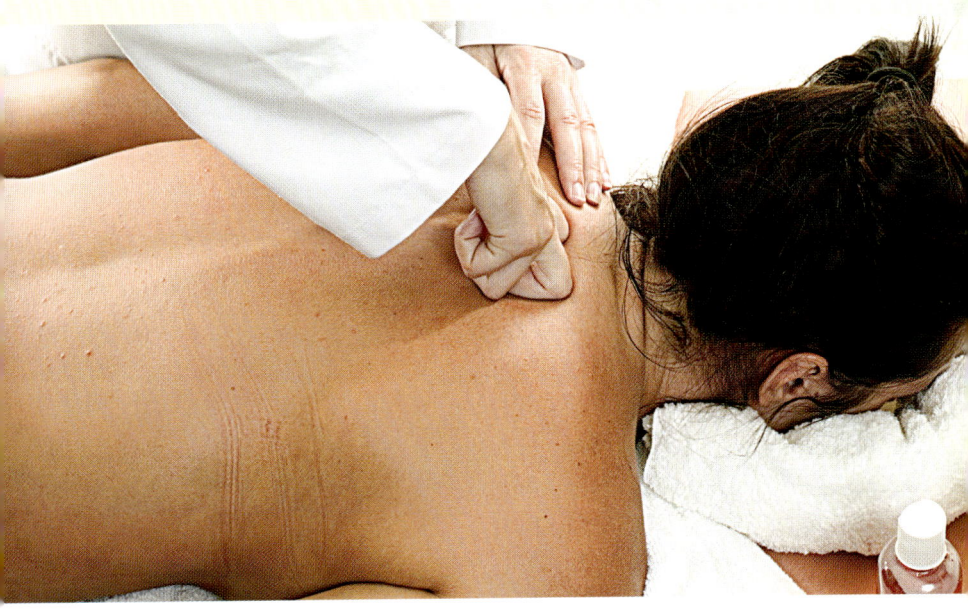

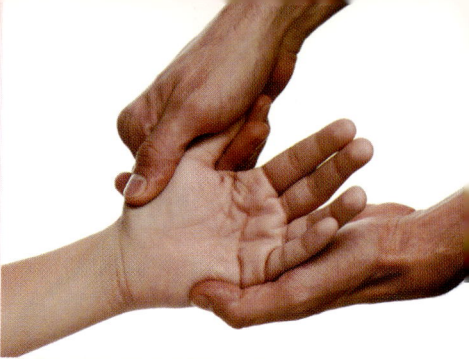

may radiate pain to other areas of the body. They can also cause muscle weakness or restricted range of motion.

Trigger points can result from a number of causes, including trauma, exposure to cold, and overuse of a muscle group.

Neuromuscular massage is a manual system of working with trigger points. Combining position and specific finger or thumb pressure into trigger or tender points in muscle and connective tissue reduce hypersensitivity, muscle spasms and referred pain patterns that characterise the point. Left untreated, such trigger points often lead to restricted and painful movement of entire body regions.

Trigger point massage is good for relieving soft tissue pain and dysfunction, improvement of circulation, pinpointing relief to specific areas. It leads to immediate relief of tension and improved muscular functioning.

Acupressure Massage

Based on the Oriental theories of energy meridians, this pressure point massage is effective in relieving tension, headaches and backaches. The focus areas are the hands, feet, face, neck, back and shoulders. No oil is used in this firm pressure massage. The session lasts for an hour.

Reflexology

This is a traditional massage employing pressure on the soles of the feet to induce deep relaxation and improve circulation. This is combined with immersion of the feet in a cool mineral bath. Ancient studies correlated the major organs, glands and body parts to specific areas of the feet. Reflexology massage manipulates these points to not only soothe the feet, but also create well-being in areas of the body.

Reflexology helps to improve blood and nerve supply, fostering a restoration of the body's natural state of equilibrium. This technique is based on the premise that the body contains energy, or 'chi', constantly flowing through channels or zones which unite to form the reflex points on the feet and hands. A session of Reflexology may last for 30 minutes.

Stone Therapy Massage

This unique therapy involves the placement of hot and cold basalt stones or marbles on strategic energy points of the body, followed by a slow, penetrating massage performed with basalt stones. The deep, penetrating heat of the volcanic basalt stones melt away the tension and stress from the body by stimulating the circulatory system and balancing the energy running through the body.

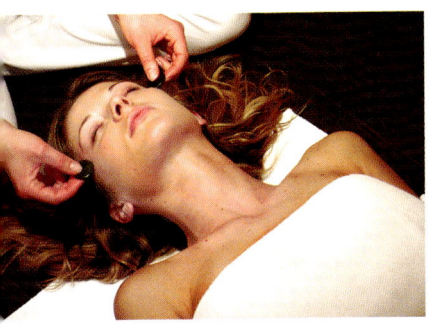

Pregnancy Massage

Pregnancy can put the body in an undue state of fatigue and lower back pressure. This specially modified massage uses a support cushion to protect the mother-to-be and her baby while the expert masseuse gently soothes her tired muscles. The massage leaves her feeling rested, pampered and stress-free, as the upper and lower back pain and aching knees get alleviated with the massage. The session may last for 50 to 80 minutes.

Craniosacral Massage

This location-directed massage is excellent for the relief of headaches, dizziness and chronic fatigue. The massage involves a very light touch and achieves excellent results. The client remains fully clothed during the session which usually lasts for an hour. Focusing on the central nervous system, the therapist deals with the bones of the head, spinal column, sacrum and underlying structures. The main objective of the work is to find restrictions and/or compression in these areas, and use specifically designed techniques to release these areas.

Lymphatic Massage

The lymphatic system is essential as the body's drainage system is cleansed and filtered out of bacteria and toxins. Congested lymph pathways can cause soreness, aches, pains and flu-like symptoms. Lymphatic massage helps to unclog the lymph system. Beginning in a clockwise motion on the body, the lymph system is manually cleansed. This massage helps the body to heal itself from many common maladies by improving the body's removal of oedemas and effusion. As with most massages, it is vital to drink lots of water after a lymphatic massage. This massage is excellent after surgery, and perfect for a very active or athletic individual who seeks a muscle intensive massage modality.

Watsu

Watsu is performed in one of the heated swimming pools in a spa. This special water technique of massage is wonderful for full-body relaxation. The client allows his body to surrender to the gentle motions of water while experiencing profound relaxation.

Chair Massage

A chair massage is, by far, the most convenient method of massage therapy. It lasts about 15 minutes. The client is seated in a specially designed chair which allows the therapist to work on the back, neck, shoulders and arms, addressing the common problem areas of today's workers. No oil is used in this massage, and the client is fully clothed.

A regular massage can reduce the physical and mental effects of stress, thus reducing burnout and stress-related diseases. A swift chair

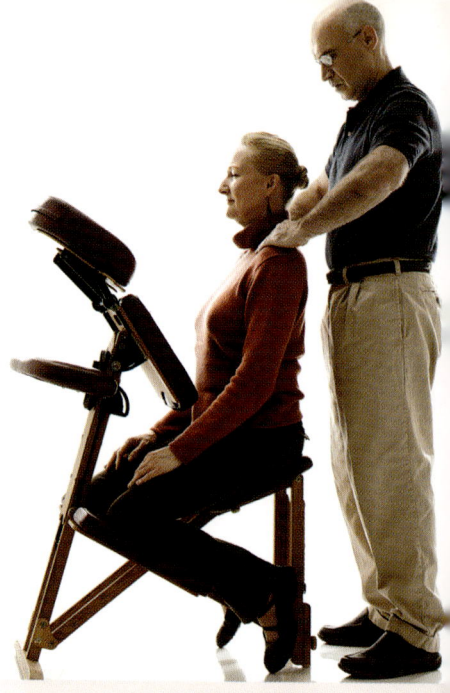

massage revitalises the anatomy, and encourages overall well-being.

Compression Massage

This is a rhythmic compression into muscles used to create a deep hyperemia and softening effect in the tissues. It is generally used as a warm-up for deeper, more specific massage work.

Punta Mita Massage

Tequila and sage form the basis of this massage. Tequila has long been known for its healing properties, and sage oil is recognised as an analgesic. Both tequila and sage have antiseptic, cleansing and detoxifying properties. The treatment begins with a relaxing hot towel application and massage to the face, abdomen and feet, to improve circulation, aid digestion and relieve the fatigue of jet-lag. This is followed by a moderately full-body massage.

Face Massage

This massage can help prevent new tension lines and wrinkles from appearing. Before starting the massage, the face is cleansed thoroughly.

Next come the basic movements – stroking, pinching and stimulating. Both hands are used to work up the neck, out across the cheeks, then gliding gently inwards, working up and over the forehead. Then a gentle pressure is applied to the temples. The skin is stimulated by the back of the therapist's hands and loosely rolling the fingers up the cheek. The skin along the jawbone is gently pinched, as also under the chin. This helps prevent a double chin. Tension around the eyes is eased by firmly squeezing the eyebrows with the thumb and forefinger. The movements are always from the bridge of the nose towards the temples. To release tension from the neck and shoulders, the therapist makes firm circular movements working up on either side of the neck, then out across the shoulders.

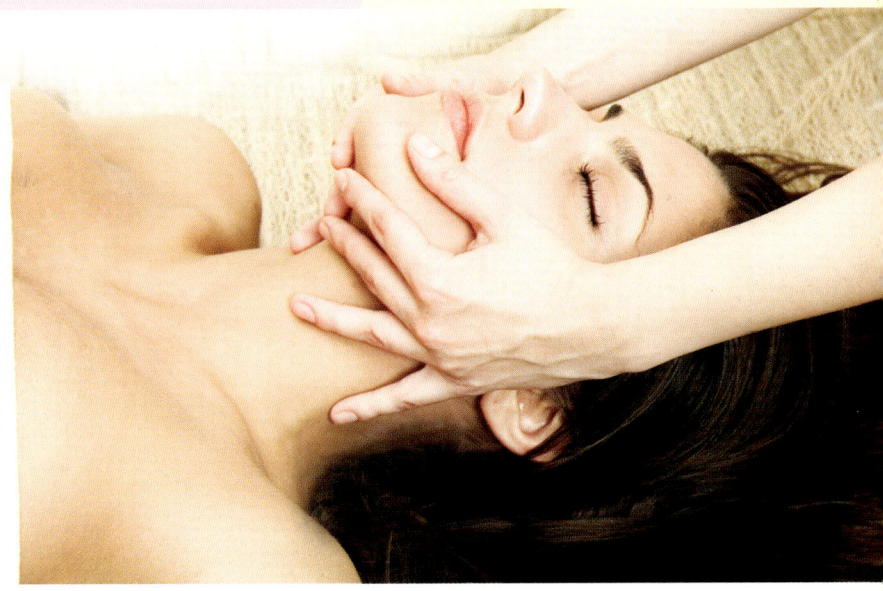

Chinese Paediatric Massage

This is a form of Tui Na massage adapted to the special needs of children up to 12 years of age. The Chinese believe that a child's energy system is different from an adult's because children have fewer physical and emotional barriers in place. Their qi is therefore more accessible to treatment. The acupoints and techniques used are different from those used with adults. A massage oil, typically sesame oil, is often used with children. The sessions are much shorter than those for adults, usually only 15-20 minutes.

Cross Fibre Massage

Friction techniques are applied in a general manner to create a stretching and broadening effect in large muscle groups. On site-specific muscle and connective tissue, deep transverse friction is applied to reduce adhesions, and to help create strong, flexible repair during the healing powers.

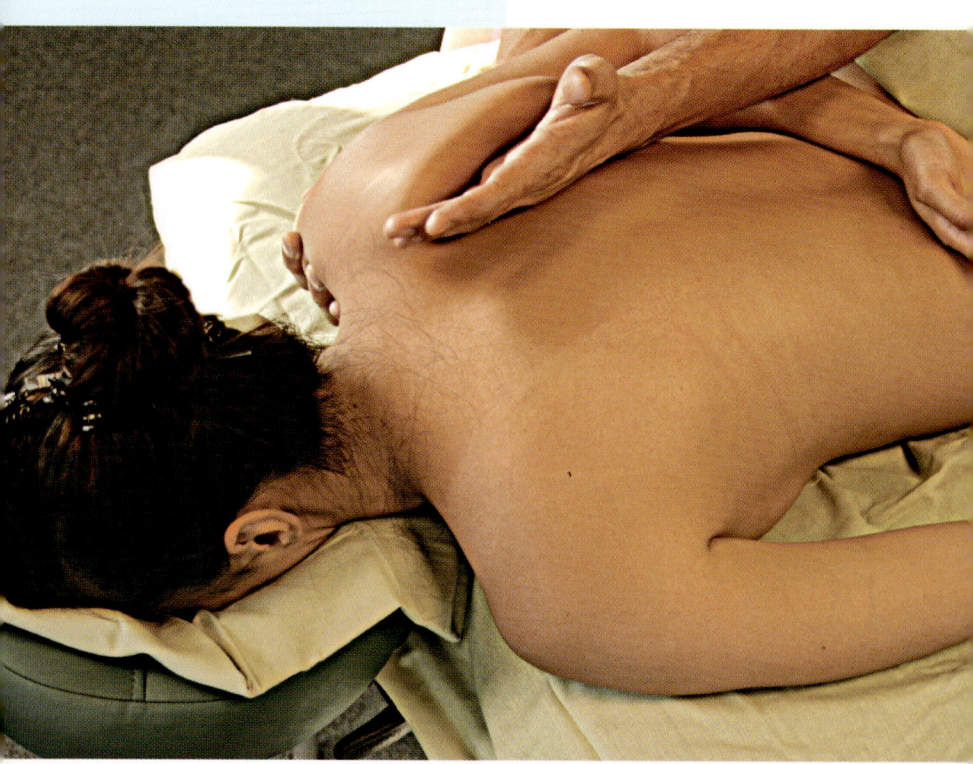

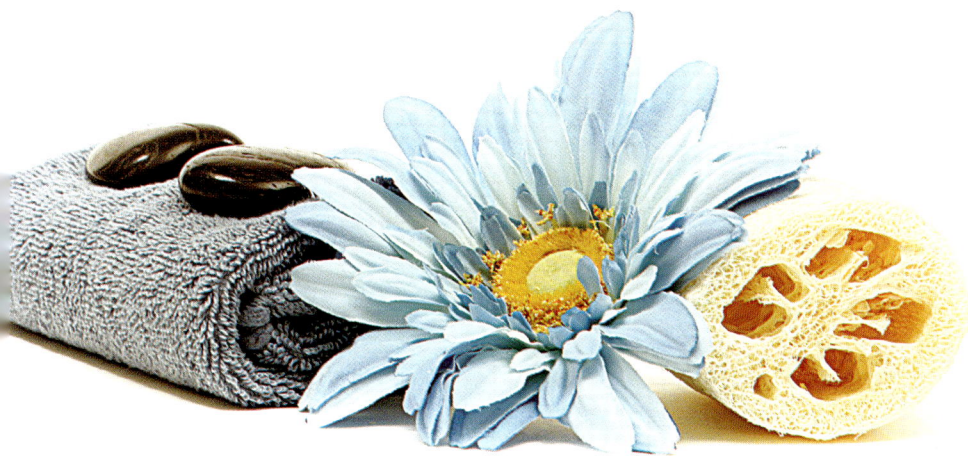

BODY SCRUBS

Regular use of a body scrub is vital for the improvement of your skin from head to toe. They work by shifting dead cells from the surface of your skin, revealing the younger, fresher ones underneath. This process also stimulates the circulation of blood in the skin tissues, giving it a rosy glow.

Most spas have their signature scrubs, but the essential ingredients are sea salts, citrus and tropical fruits, honey, milk, oatmeal, coconut, flowers, clay and mud, herbs, minerals and sugar.

Some of the more common scrubs used in spas the world over are given as follows.

Lulur Jimbaran

Kur Lulur Jimbaran combines a Javanese beauty ritual and the ultimate in pampering. It begins with a relaxing Balinese massage, followed by exfoliation with granular turmeric, sandalwood, rice powder, herbal wood, ginger root and spices. This is finished off with a yoghurt splash to neutralise the skin. Then you are allowed to soak in a bath infused with flowers.

Aromatherapy Ancient Sea Salt Scrub

The ancient sea salts provide an invaluable source of nutrients and trace minerals to the skin. They are blended with pure aromatherapy oils for an exfoliating treatment. You can choose between relaxing sea salts or stimulating sea salts. It gives a new radiance to your skin.

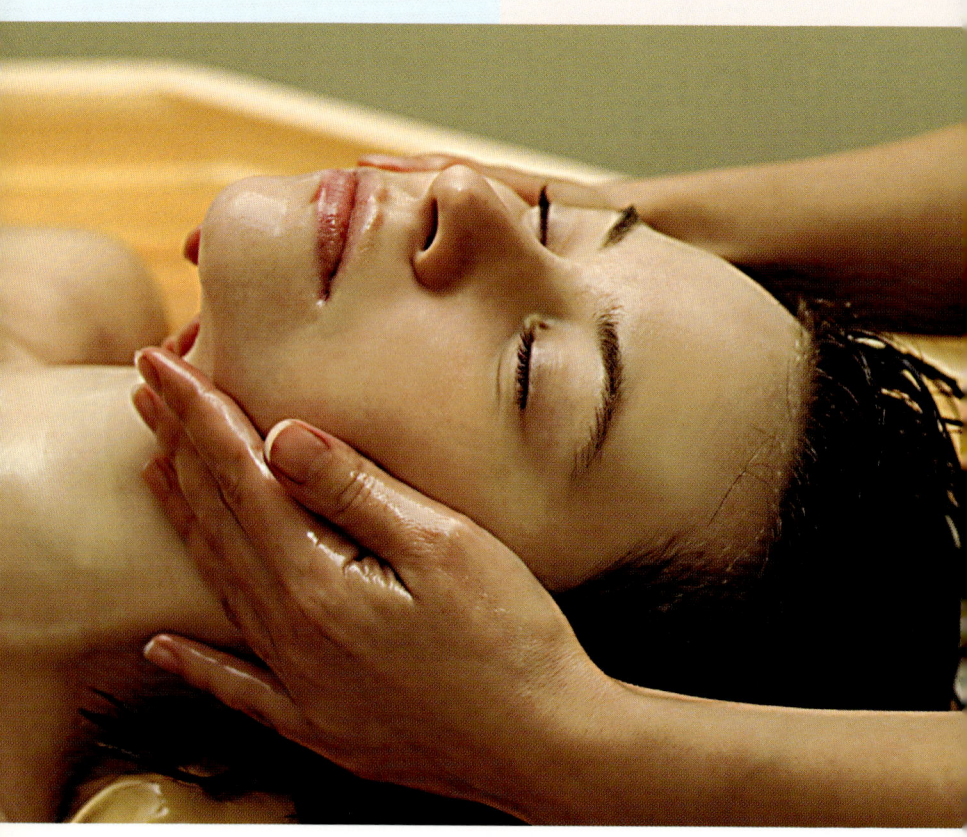

Aromatherapy and Hydro Massage Scrub

This is a multi-step treatment beginning with a body exfoliation using olive grains and your choice of aromatherapy body wash followed by a luxurious soak in a thalasso tub filled with filtered sea water and bath essential oils.

Sea Salt Body Scrub

Warm oils and pure salt are applied all over the body for a de-stressing and nourishing treatment designed to release toxins from the skin. This full-body exfoliation will help the skin to be radiant and glowing.

Dead Sea Salt Scrub

Some body scrubs are concocted with exotic salts, such as those from the Dead Sea which is known for its rich minerals and healing properties. This premium treatment leaves your skin soft, and the body and mind feeling refreshed and invigorated.

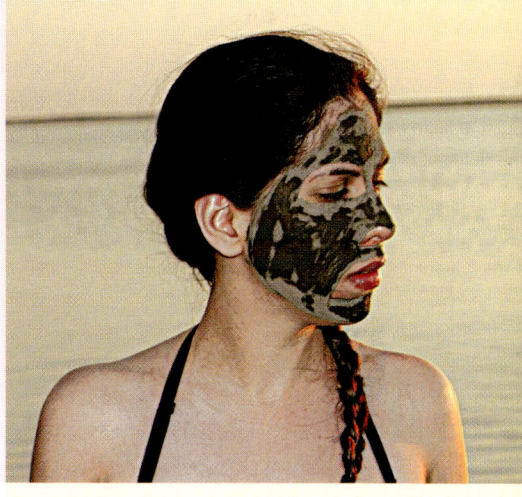

Turkish Salt Scrub

An invigorating thermal mineral salt exfoliation applied in a two-step treatment, utilising thermal salt, rich in minerals and trace elements, followed by a loofah scrub with thermal mineral shower.

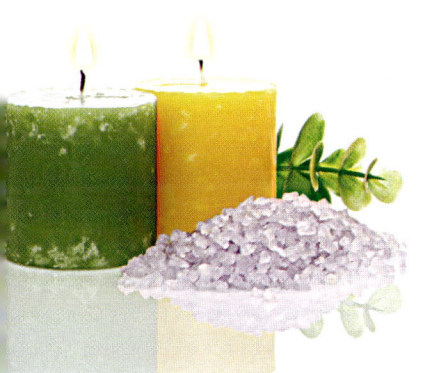

Balinese Boreh

This is a traditional Balinese special scrub made from indigenous ingredients including some hot spices as cloves, pepper, nutmeg, cardamom, ginger and galangal.

Italian Fango Therapy

A rich moor mud combined with paraffin is heated and applied as a localised heat pack to a stressed and tensed area such as the neck and shoulders, the lower back, or stiff joints.

Loofah Scrub

The body is cleaned and scrubbed with a loofah mitt and seaweed shower gel, promoting circulation.

Mandarin Orange and Brown Sugar Scrub

This is an exceptional full-body exfoliation, using extracts of mandarin orange and brown sugar. This treatment smoothens, softens and enriches the skin, leaving it looking fresh and tingling.

Papaya Enzyme Scrub

Made with a gel, papaya and natural ingredients, this scrub gently exfoliates the skin and softens it.

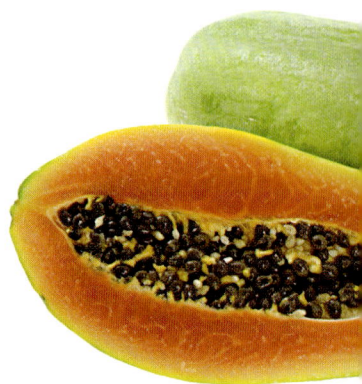

Avocado Scrub

Fresh avocado, honey and rice powder are rich in vitamins. They are combined with natural oil and used as an effective scrub to soften a dry and sun-exposed skin.

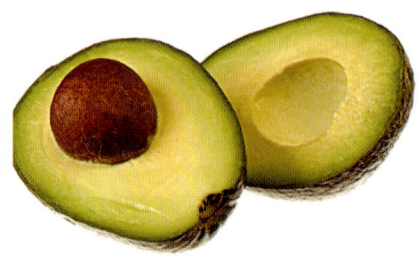

Coconut Scrub

Coconut is naturally rich in oil, and therefore freshly grated coconut is a gentle scrub for nourishing dry or sensitive skin.

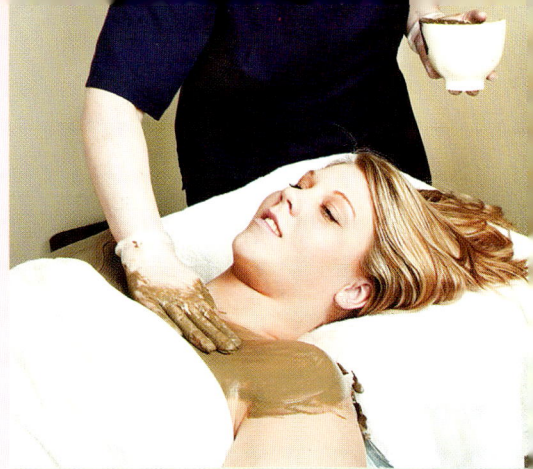

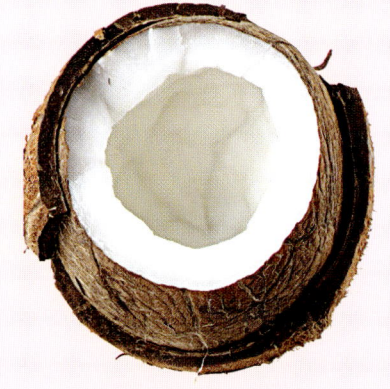

Seaweed Scrub

Seaweed is a ocean's gift to health and beauty! It has high mineral and trace element content which stimulates the metabolism and speeds up the elimination of toxins.

Body Mud and Salt Scrub

The combination of herbal body mud and salt scrub has a full cleansing and detoxification effect on the body, which will leave you looking radiant and feeling wonderful.

▼ Lotus Body Scrub

The natural secrets of the lotus plant, an aquatic herb, help slow the ageing process. It rejuvenates your skin by promoting exfoliation and removing impurities. A lotion massage buffs the skin into a healthy, radiant and beautiful glow.

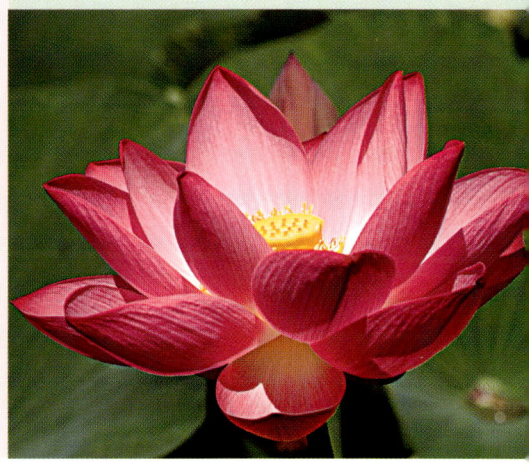

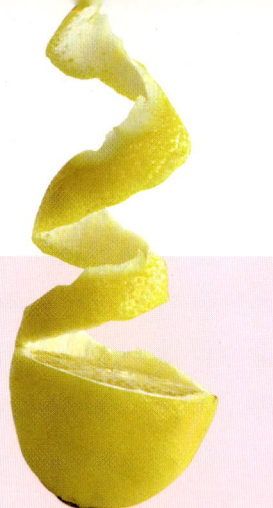

☑ Lime Refresher Scrub

Lime peel gives this scrub its delightful fresh scent, and at the same time acts as an antiseptic. It is mixed with wheat germ and honey. The latter softens and nourishes the skin while the former heals and smoothens out lines with its rich vitamin E content.

☑ Turmeric-Honey Scrub

This scrub is renowned for its healing and cleansing properties. Turmeric is mixed with honey, tamarind and sesame seeds to make it a refreshing scrub for all skin types. The oil from the crushed sesame seeds ensures that the skin is not stripped dry by the scrub.

☑ Tropical Fruit Scrub

Banana, papaya, watermelon, pineapple and orange are used in this exotic and natural exfoliant that softens and clears the skin as it cleanses and tightens the pores.

☑ Coffee Body Scrub

The magnificent aroma and natural qualities of coffee grains are the perfect carrier of this delicious exfoliation.

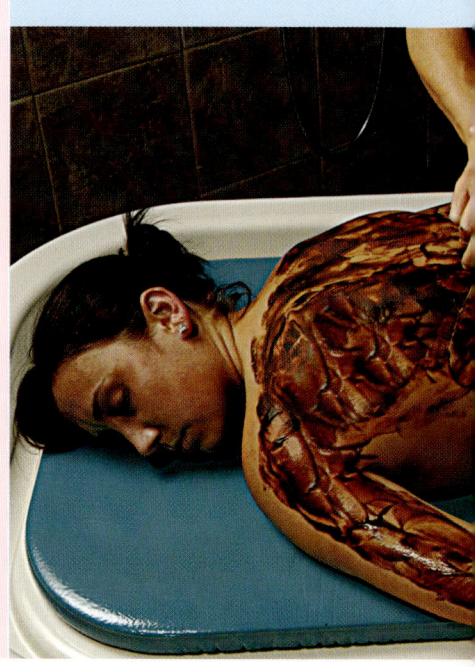

Fruity Body Scrub

A concoction of apricot pits and strawberries makes an excellent scrub that leaves your skin silky smooth and glowing.

Herbal Scrub

A mixture of traditional herbs with honey and sesame seeds is used as a body scrub to cleanse and remove dead skin cells. It moisturises and encourages new cell growth to produce a healthier skin.

Blended Brush Scrub

This scrub consists of oatmeal, fresh milk, honey, tamarind and watermelon. It will remove dead skin cells and replenish moisture for a softer and smoother skin.

Citrus Sugar Scrub

Citrus is combined with sugar for this delightful scrub. Citrus is offered as a natural glycolic and essential oil to increase exfoliation.

Green Tea Body Glow

Green tea has been regarded for centuries as powerful antioxidant. This is a gentle exfoliant, using jojoba to delicately buff away the dead skin cells, leaving the skin feeling refreshed and radiant looking.

Orange Scrub

This luscious citrus-based scrub uses the oranges of Florida along with healing oils, fragrant oranges and rose petal essence to soften your skin.

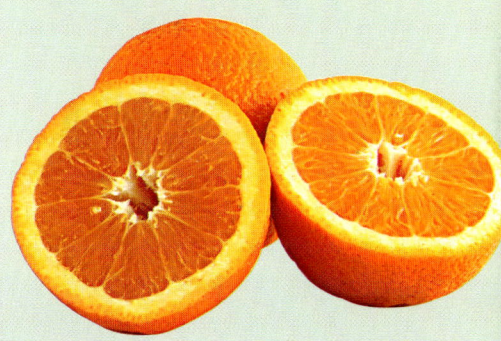

Grape Scrub

Your pampering begins with a full-body grape seed scrub with rosemary and herbal flowers to smooth out and exfoliate the skin.

Vanilla Body Scrub

Mineral-rich sea salts combined with natural herbs and essential oils are used to exfoliate and nourish your skin. Natural extracts of apricot and avocado, Dead Sea salts and pure vanilla combine to rejuvenate your skin.

Peppermint-Rosemary Scrub

Peppermint, rosemary and Dead Sea salts with vitamin E invigorate and bring a glow to your skin.

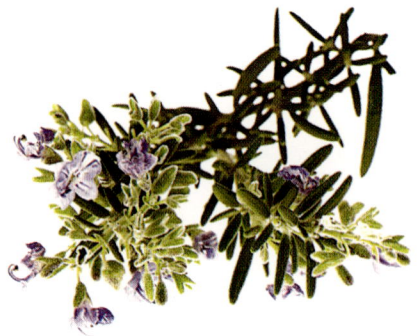

Tangerine Body Scrub

Tangerine, sweet orange, essential oils, Dead Sea salts, nourishing vitamin E and apricot exfoliate and nourish your skin.

Tropical Skin Scrub

Sea water crystals are blended with lavender, lemon grass and nutmeg oil for skin conditioning and overall health. This scrub is a dynamic way to increase circulation, exfoliate the skin and mildly detoxify the body.

Chamomile Body Scrub

The body is gently exfoliated with a soothing chamomile body polish. A chamomile gel loofah scrub and chamomile dry oil spray leave you feeling fully revitalised.

Hibiscus-Papaya Scrub

This is a soothing, non-abrasive body scrub. It consists of papaya enzymes and the natural antioxidants supplied from vitamin C-rich hibiscus flowers.

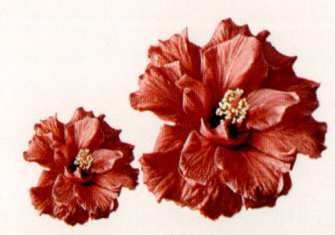

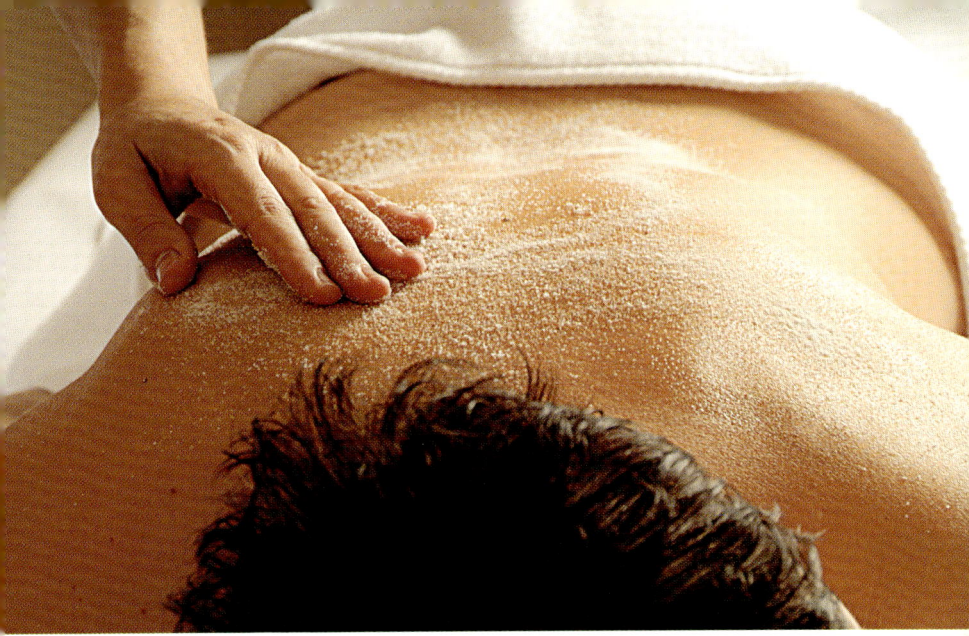

BODY WRAPS and POLISHES

SPAS

Body wraps have been used for centuries for their deeply relaxing benefits to the body and mind as well as for detoxification and relief from water retention. Every body wrap includes a vigorous dry brushing to loosen dry skin and stimulate the lymphatic system, and a finishing massage at the conclusion of the treatment. After a scrub or body wrap, your skin is pampered with essential oils and aloe vera, polishing off with a scented bath.

Some of the more common body wraps that are available in most of the spas are given as follows.

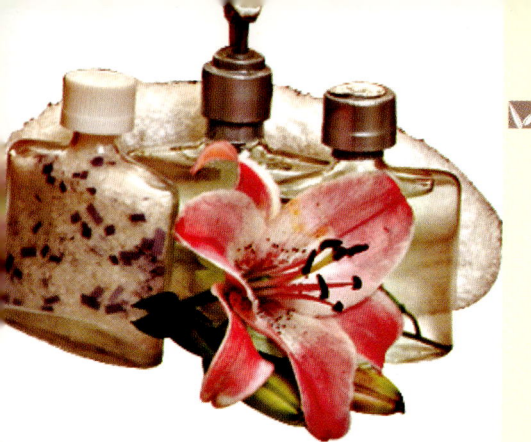

Balinese Boreh Wrap

Deeply warmed spices like clove, ginger, pepper and nutmeg create a warming wrap for the body, thus stimulating and rejuvenating your tired body.

Aromatherapy Oil Wrap

This deep moisturising treatment begins with a gentle dry brushing. A soothing full-body wrap, using synergistically blended oils combined with an aromatherapy oil of your choice, such as relaxing lavender or reviving grapefruit, will leave your skin tingling and glowing with freshness.

Aloe Wrap

Healing aloe is generously applied to your skin. While you are snugly wrapped, enjoy some scalp massage or facial. This wrap is completed with a coconut-butter application that leaves the body soothed, softened and hydrated.

Aloe-Lavender Body Wrap

Hydrating and luxurious fresh aloe vera gel and soothing lavender are applied to the skin, then wrapped in banana leaves to cool and soothe the body. This wrap is excellent for reconditioning and regenerating sunburned skin. It finishes with an application of lavender lotion moisturiser.

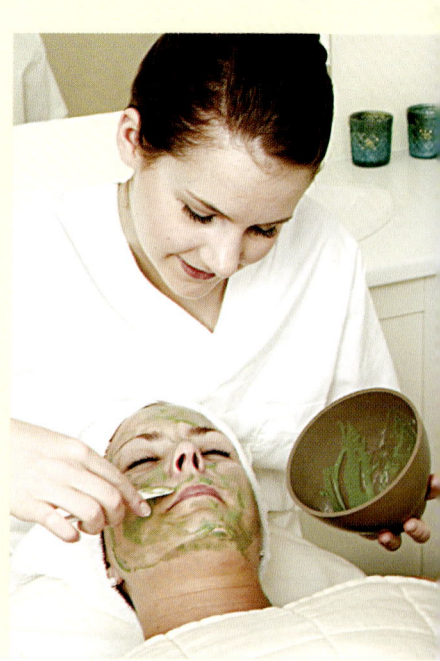

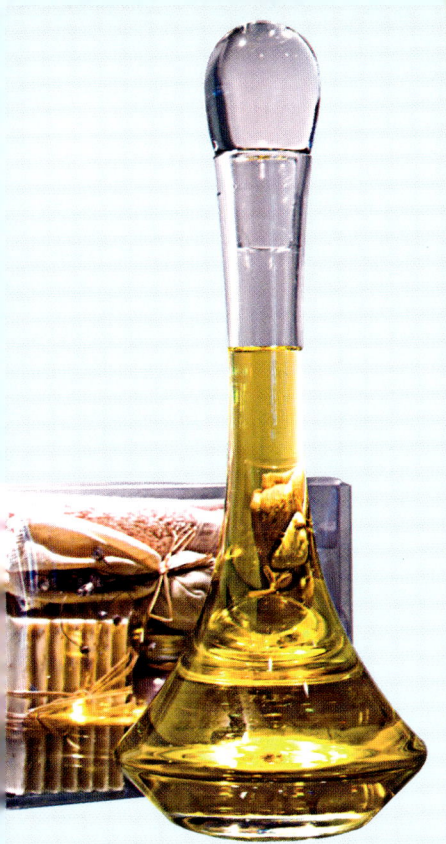

Sea Body Mask

Rich seaweed skin and body care lotion is applied on the body for revitalising and toning. The high mineral and trace-element content stimulates the metabolism, and temporarily reduces water retention.

Natural Spirulina Wrap

This wrap envelops you in an all-natural spirulina algae that is nourishing, stimulating and revitalising for the body. Spirulina is rich in proteins, vitamins and minerals which will promote healthy radiant-looking skin.

Lavender Wrap

After the body is scrubbed and exfoliated, it is misted with sandalwood paste to balance the skin. Then wild lavender emulsion is used on the body to further enhance healing and restoration. The treatment is completed with an application of peppermint glycolic cream to stimulate the skin while cooling and closing the pores, leaving your skin healthy and radiant.

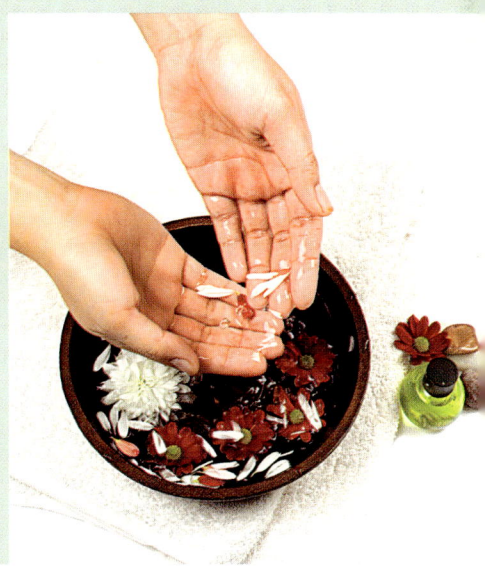

Dead Sea Body Wrap

The healing properties of the Dead Sea have been recognised for many years. Known for its purification benefits, this body wrap will leave your skin feeling clean and refreshed. A rich cream is massaged into the skin to complete the treatment.

Herbal Wrap

Towels steamed in pure chamomile, rose petals and lavender are placed on the body. Sheets and blankets are used to encase the moist, scented warmth. This treatment promotes relaxation and the release of toxins through perspiration. This treatment is excellent for stress reduction.

Sea Water Aromatherapy Wrap

This sea water-based body wrap with the therapeutic essential oils of basil, lavender, sage, sandalwood and ylang-ylang is superb for those enduring stress and fatigue. It provides remineralisation, improves micro-circulation, and stimulates cellular regeneration.

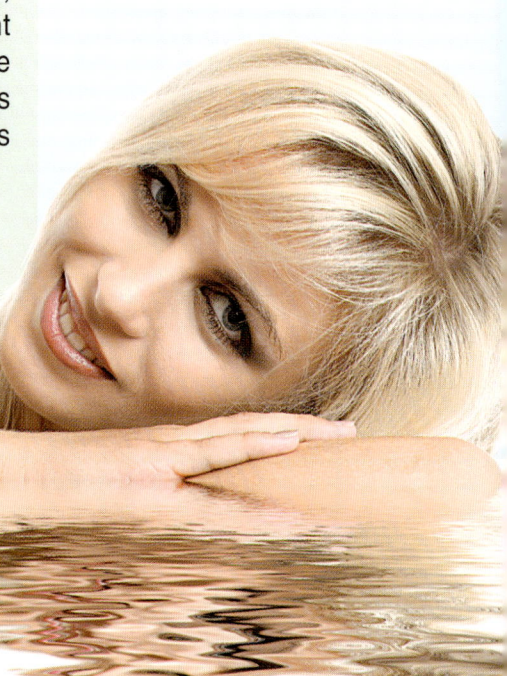

Milk-Honey Rehydrating Wrap

The milk and honey body wrap is a maximum performance-conditioning and revitalising body wrap – ideal to indulge and regenerate body skin. Lactic acid eliminates dry and rough spots; vitamins and trace elements activate skin metabolism. Skin balance is restored, and it instantly imports a velvety soft skin.

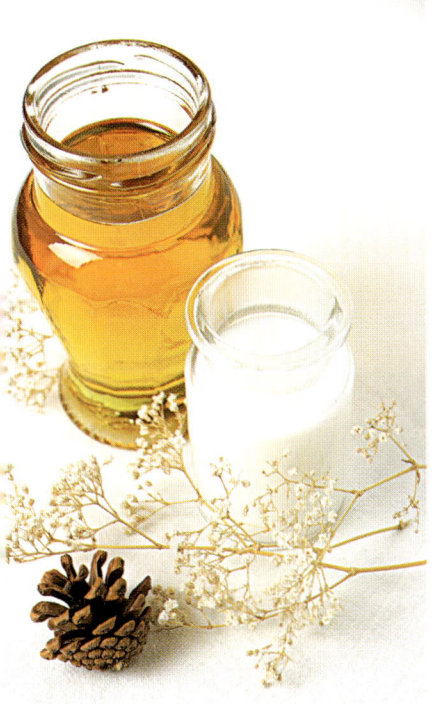

Mud Wrap

Your body will be masked in dark mineral clay, thus remineralising your skin, while absorbing impurities and improving its oxygen supply. You will be wrapped in a heated blanket to aid in the mineral absorption, and then cleansed in a warm shower to emerge with a soft pure skin and a relaxed mind.

Moor Mud Wrap

The healing and rejuvenating properties of 'Moor Mud' have been known since ancient times. This mud is found in only a few select places in the world, and is known to have over thousands of healing herbs and minerals. This detoxifying and purifying warm mud is applied

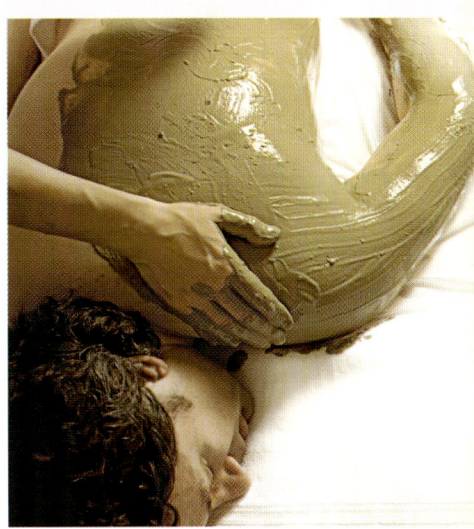

to the body following a light brushing of the skin. A warm towel wrap is followed by a quick shower and application of hydrating lotion.

Hibiscus Clay Mask

This purifies the body with mineral-rich mud from the earth, scented with the delightful smell of hibiscus flowers.

Chocolate Wrap

The chocolate wrap is used as an exfoliation and hydration cream.

The lactic acids in the milk bring the toxins to the surface of the skin, so they are washed away. The skin becomes clear and radiant.

Micro Body Buff Polish

This skin exfoliation technique uses buffing beads, apricot powder, wheat, amino acids and lactic acids to penetrate the epidermis which attracts and locks in moisture, accelerates epidermal cell renewal, and lifts away surface dryness. You will love this if you have a mature or sensitive skin.

Acti-Sea Body Mud Wrap

This is a very effective treatment for smoothing, stimulating and detoxifying the skin and body. Acti-sea body mud contains a potent mix of five French seaweeds and marine actives to stimulate, firm and moisturise the skin.

Algae Body Polish

This is a gentle exfoliation, recommended especially for

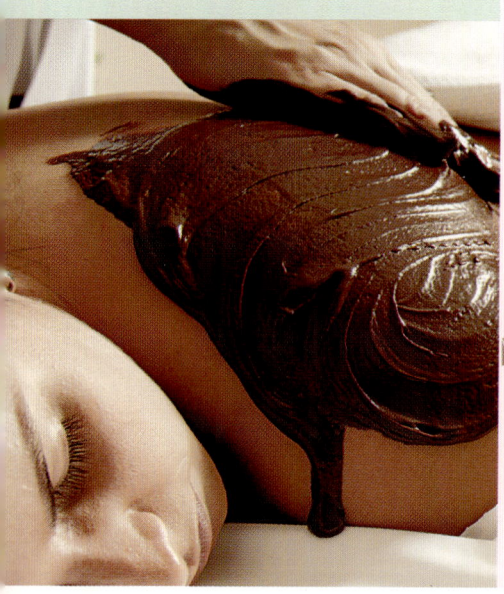

sensitive skin, using the exfoliating benefits of unicellular algae and the moisturising of pine oil.

Shea Butter Wrap

Shea butter is mixed with lavender essential oil to help promote restful sleep and deep relaxation. The treatment starts with a dry brush to the body, and then the butter is applied with long massage strokes. After the application of butter, the entire body of the guest or client will be wrapped in a warm cocoon, and given a head and foot massage.

Fruit Extract Body Polish

The natural peel of lemons and oranges exfoliates the skin, while the scent of the fruits is awakening and invigorating.

Apres Sun Recovery Wrap

This is a perfect antidote that is sensitive and overexposed to the sun. It is gentle enough for even the sunburnt skin. This wrap has active ingredients like aloe, green algae, green tea and calming lavender which are used to help restore hydration and reduce redness.

Papaya-Passion Fruit Body Mask

It is a body mask of clay that is imbued with the enzymes of papaya and passion fruit, and natural fruit acids which rehydrate and retexture the skin during a detoxifying body wrap.

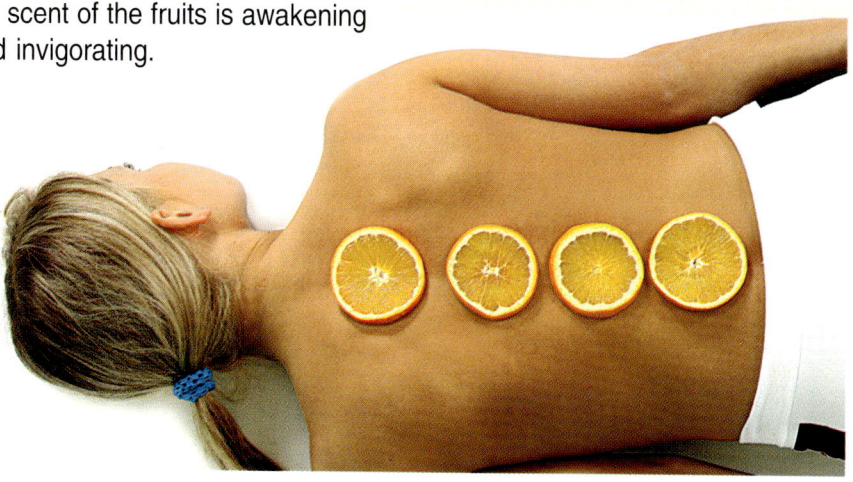

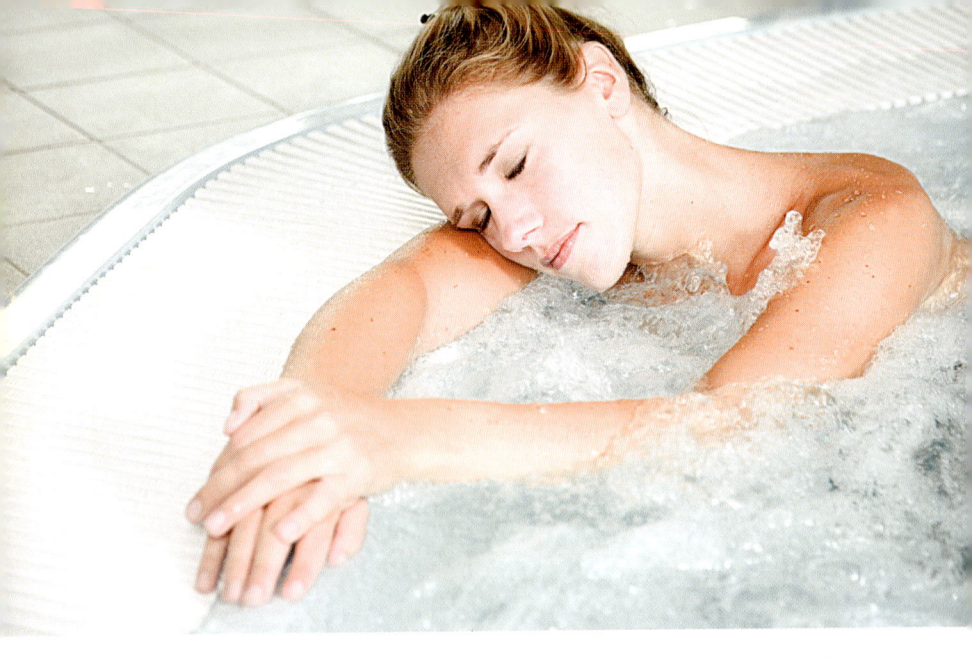

INVIGORATING
BATHS

SPAS

Caring for your body creates endless rewards. These days, spas offer the whole gamut of shower gels, bubble baths, bath oils and salts, and aromatic herbs. Soaking in a warm bath with fragrant and invigorating salts and gels has to be one of the most popular ways to relax.

Bath time can become an aromatherapy treat when essential oils such as chamomile and lavender are added to the water. Just add a few drops in your bath, then lie back, inhale the fragrance and vapours, and relax. Salts and bubble baths that contain sea minerals and kelp also have a relaxing and purifying effect on the body and skin, respectively.

Cider Vinegar Bath

This bath helps to tauten the flabby skin, and remove the toxins that may be embedded in the top layer of the skin.

Epsom Salt Bath

This bath helps to neutralise the acid waste materials in the body tissue. The salts also help to open clogged pores, and eliminate toxins.

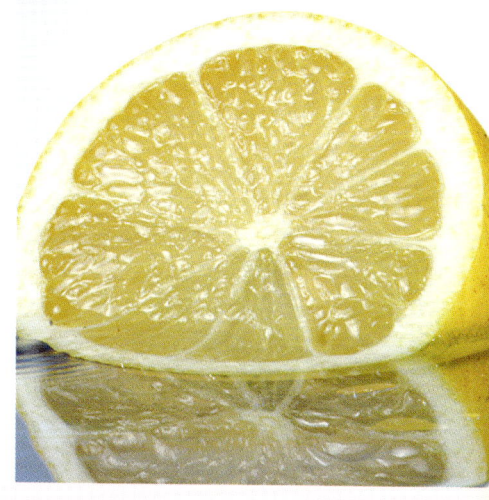

☑ Lemon Bath

A few lemon peels along with lemon juice and aromatic herbs leave your skin glowing and tingling.

☑ Aroma Steam Bath

The sequence begins with hydrotherapy in your private aromatic steam room, with a choice of lavender-eucalyptus or lemon grass-mint essential oils, alternating with refreshing dips in your own pool. Following this invigorating regime, you are pampered with a lotion massage of your choice, using the same essential oils as the hydrotherapy session. It is an excellent way to improve breathing, promote internal and external body relaxation, and awaken the senses. It is also a perfect remedy for jet lag.

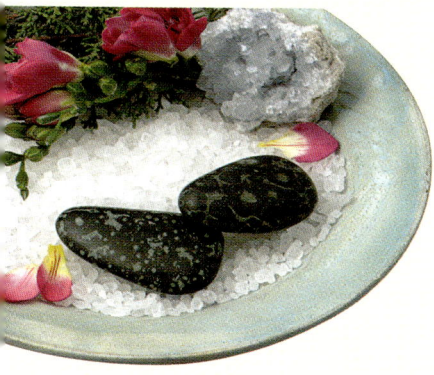

Milk Bath

Having this bath is an ideal way to nourish and soften the skin. Some spas add oatmeal powder, rose petals and a few drops of almond oil in the milk bath to rejuvenate dull skins.

Garden Bath

Tropical flower petals and leaves are combined with exotic lavender, ylang-ylang and bergamot to create a soothing bath experience.

Thalassotherapy

It is a treatment with the rejuvenating effects of the sea to help relax and nourish the body. Immerse yourself in a seaweed bath infused with eucalyptus oil, and then finish with a luxurious massage using marine lotion and firming cream.

Sea Algae Bath

This treatment is an ideal way to relax and nourish the body. First, you are gently cocooned in warm spirulina algae, allowing your skin to soak in the valuable antioxidants. Next, you are immersed in a bath laden with sea salts and sea algae. After that a luxurious massage with lavender and mineral cream completes this deluxe treatment.

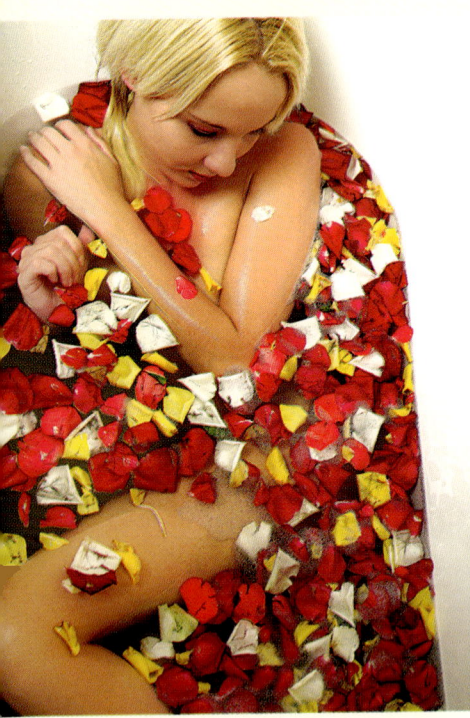

Thermal Bath

Relax in your private hydrotherapy suite, and soak for 15 minutes in a bubbly hot tub with aromatic scents that will benefit tight muscles and reduce stress. You have the choice of thermal mineral or aromatherapy oils.

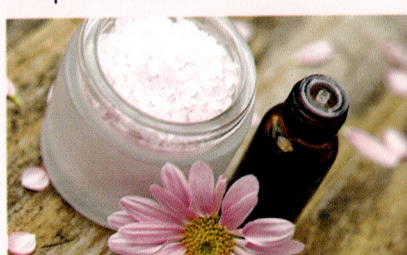

Herbal Bath

Relax in a herbal bath that contains pine and essential oils. After the bath, experience a luxurious massage with lavender essential oil.

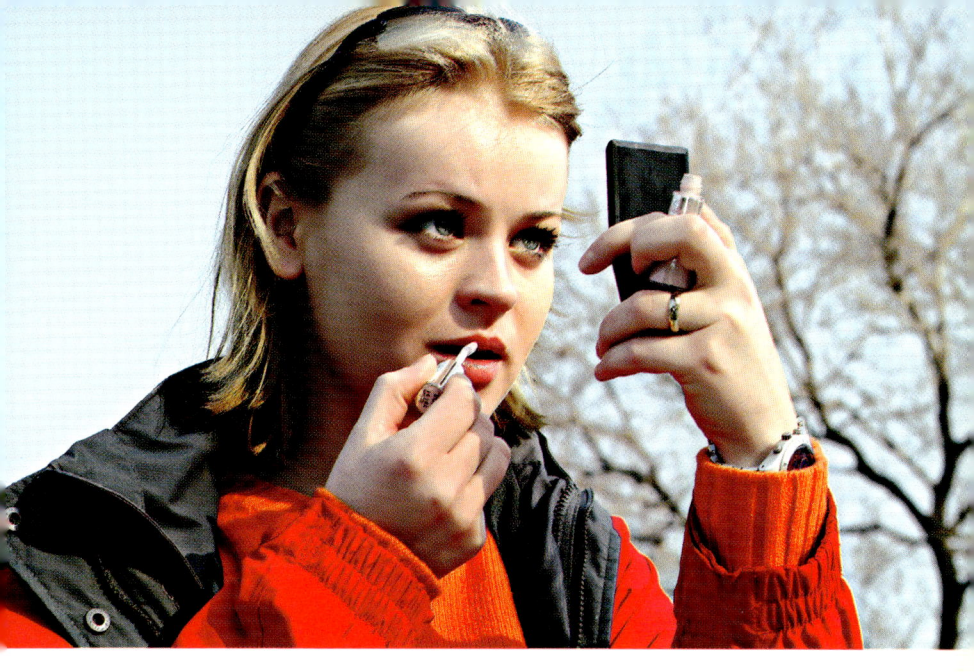

BEAUTY
TREATMENTS

A luxurious facial is a great way to restore the glow to a weary, parched skin. And these days, spas offer a wide selection of facials: from anti-ageing to aromatherapy. Deep cleansing, extra-hydrating, anti-ageing, acne treatment, exfoliation, massage and mask are included in beauty treatments.

Since face care is the most important part of beauty care, most spas focus on this aspect of beauty treatment, giving a golden glow to your face. Normally, spas offer a long list of face care treatments for you to select from.

Given ahead are some of the more common facials offered at various spas.

SPAS

Thai Honey Facial

This is ideal for a sunburnt and sensitive skin, and designed where exfoliation is not recommended. This treatment provides a light cleansing followed by a gentle and relaxing facial massage using honey. A hydrating fresh cucumber mask completes the facial, restoring balance.

Sari Jimbaran Facial

This is a facial mask with essences of natural botanicals, tropical ylang-ylang flowers and potpourri, combined with beneficial aromatherapy and modern herbal formulations.

Four-layer Facial

This is a facial for all skin types. This famous facial uses the elements of the sea to create dramatic results. The first layer consists of a seaweed filtrate from freshly harvested seaweed to rebalance and tone skin tissue. The second layer is a hydrating cream and facial massage. The third one is a fresh seaweed mask to eliminate toxins and nourish cells. Layer four is the self-heating mineral mask made to activate the properties of the seaweed mask beneath it.

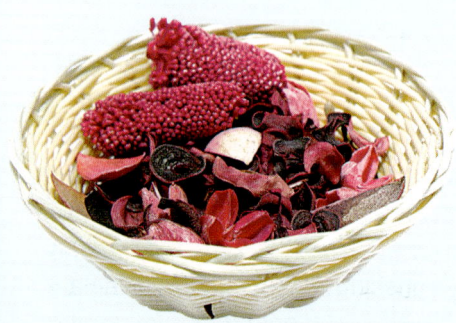
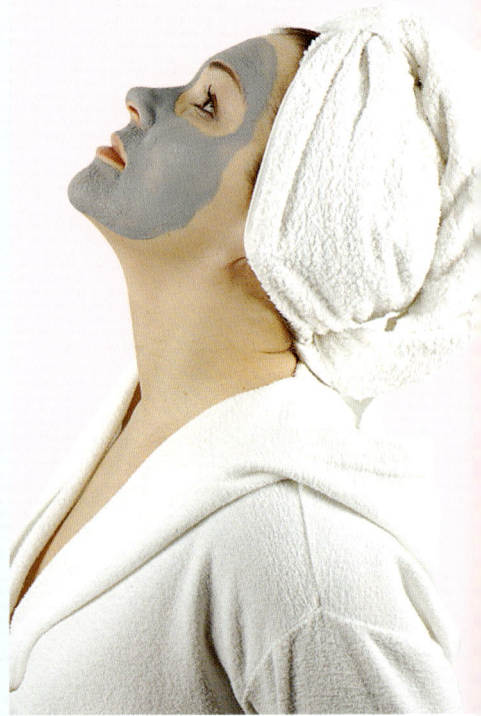

Essensa Anti-stress Facial

This French aromatherapy uses pure essential oils to treat tired, stressed skin. The facial includes cleansing, exfoliation, gel mask, hydrating fruit mask, and a special facial massage to relax, rehydrate and revitalise the skin.

Japanese Facial

This is an energising technique used to stimulate acupressure points through the lifting and toning of the face and scalp. This is believed to have a cumulative effect when used on a regular basis for firming the skin and preserving a youthful appearance.

Absolute Hydration Facial

This facial consists of custom-blended cleansers and moisturisers, and a mask of natural plant extracts, giving you a fresh, radiant complexion—with three levels of response designed to treat young, over-indulged or extremely dehydrated skin.

Aloe-Lavender Facial

This is a cooling and refreshing facial, especially for a sunburnt skin, with a revitalising mask, aloe vera gel and lavender essential oil.

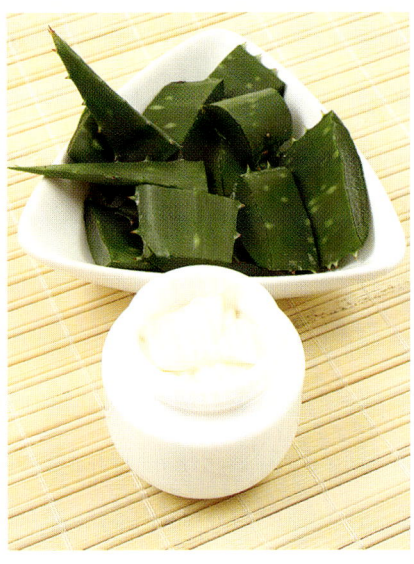

Revitalising Facial

This is beneficial for a mature and dry skin. This deep hydration treatment has been specially designed to bring freshness, vitality and glow to a tired and dry skin. A nourishing mask is used to stimulate the skin, prevent premature ageing and reduce signs of tiredness.

☑ Balancing Facial for Oily Skin

This is an enzyme-based facial that controls oily secretions by reducing the flow of sebum and balancing the skin's pH. It virtually eliminates all bacteria and leaves the skin fresh and matte.

☑ Papaya Enzyme Peel Facial

Papaya and enzymes join together to create a highly effective exfoliant, specially designed to fight fine lines and blemishes.

☑ European Seaweed Facial

Natural ingredients from the sea and the purest marine extracts are used in this facial. Your skin is gently cleansed with a sea enzyme cleanser, followed by a soothing massage, then finishing with a cooling and refreshing sea enzyme focus, coral plus C mask or an enzyme seaweed mask that is suitable for all skin types.

☑ Replenishing Facial

This facial is an intense oxygenating programme to arouse tired, stressed and asphyxiated skin. It makes the skin luminous and refreshed by employing aromatherapy and a mask made of natural fruit extracts and vitamins.

☑ Oxygen Activator Facial

It is good for sallow, tired-looking skin. The oxygen is designed to give your tired and sallow skin a jump-start. After cleansing, toning and exfoliating, your face is covered with two masks. First, an activator mask is applied to help firm the skin, then an oxygen mask is applied for 20 minutes. After that a facial massage with an essential oil concludes the treatment, leaving behind a soft and nourished skin.

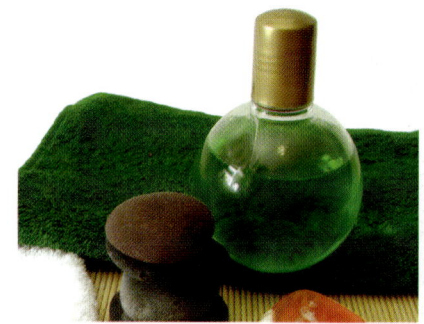

Aromatherapy Facial

It is a soothing, hydrating facial for a dry and normal skin. A mask with roses, geranium and jasmine essential oils will provide immediate luminosity and radiance to your skin.

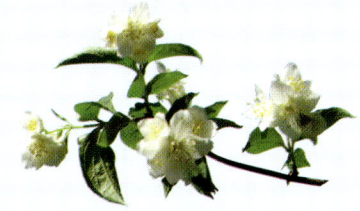

Aromatherapy Purifying Facial

In this facial, pure honey, oatmeal and almond scrub are mixed with fresh buttermilk to gently exfoliate the dead skin cells, followed by extraction, and then a mask to promote healing and reduce oiliness. This is the perfect facial with custom-blend purifying and calming essential oils to leave an oily or combination skin super clean and healthy.

Sea Breeze Facial

It is great for a sensitive skin. The exclusive green tea and ginger mask deeply cleanses to soften the skin and refine enlarged pores so that the skin appears even and smooth.

Cold Marine Facial

This cold marine mask has a tightening effect which smooths out and relaxes stress lines. This facial encourages vasoconstriction and stimulation of facial blood circulation.

Golden Spoons Facial

This is a facial utilising 23 carat-plated spoons where one is hot (actually warm when touched) and the other is cold. The facialist applies alternately each one to generate efficacious penetration of the creams and lotions, and also to open and close pores, stimulating circulation.

Men's Marine Facial

Men often take their skin for granted, not giving it the attention it needs, thus it can become dry and irritated by shaving and exposure to sun, humidity or harsh, dry weather. The marine facial soothes the over-shaved, over-stressed face, reduces razor burn and redness, and helps eliminate the occurrence of ingrown hairs. It provides an invigorating massage; warm, deep pore steaming; a cleansing scrub; and a reviving mask followed by a brisk toner and a refreshing moisturiser.

Beta-A Complex Facial

This is very good for oily skin or blemish-prone complexions. Following an antibacterial cleansing and toning, an alpha-hydroxy acid exfoliating cream and Tazorac (a prescription oil-reducing and pore-minimising treatment) are left on the face for 20 minutes. After clogged-pore extractions and a massage, a layer of a non-comedogenic moisturiser completes the facial.

Corrective Care Facial

This special treatment detoxifies, oxygenates and invigorates skin cells by using benzoyl peroxide, enzyme peel and a mask designed to draw away toxins in acne-prone skin. A separate mask is then used to soothe and heal your skin. A pro-biotic cream combined with aloe vera is used to hydrate and heal your treated skin.

Oxyliance Cellular Facial

Oxyliance breathes a bubble of fresh air into the skin, leaving it feeling hydrated, pure and beautiful. Its unique, pollution-combating formula gives radiance and vitality to the skin. It also lightens the complexion and adds a sparkle and freshness to the face.

Ayurveda Facial

This is a great treatment that employs 100 per cent pure aromatherapy oil which is infused into the skin via gentle massage and warm compresses. The massage, using acupressure and stroking techniques, covers the upper body. A refreshing mask follows.

Wrinkle Control Facial

The signs of ageing skin fade away with this facial which consist of active ingredients like aloe vera, collagen, elastin, and hyaluronic acid that are capable of reducing the depth of wrinkles by an instant smoothing effect.

Vitamin C - Oxygen Facial

Oxygen is vital for healthy and youthful looking skin. This mask is a powerful tool to keep the oxygen active against the skin, while temporarily preventing it from evaporating. Oxygenating the surface of the skin with a combination of vitamin-C complex essential oils is an activating treatment with a phenomenal result.

ACE Antioxidant Facial

This is an excellent facial for all skin types, using antioxidant vitamins A, C and E (ACE). This treatment helps revitalise a stressed, sun-damaged and environmentally-damaged skin. This facial includes an extra-relaxing facial massage and thermal modelling mask.

AHA Flash Facial

A skin-revitalising facial treatment with alpha hydroxy acids accelerates the removal of dry dead surface cells, contributing to a finer, clearer complexion. After cleansing the face, a gentle AHA facial serum and mask application will contribute to a more refined skin texture and smoother appearance.

Sunburn Treatment

This treatment has been specifically designed to rejuvenate tired and damaged skin with the purest essential oil compress and purifying mask. It soothes your burnt body with aloe vera gel.

Glycolic Facial

This is perfect for a deep exfoliation, and the glycolic treatment will help to refine texture, minimise the appearance of fine lines and promote a balanced skin tone.

Vitamin C Facial

This is a highly effective antioxidant treatment that delivers immediate results. L-asorbic acid (vitamin C) helps smooth the skin as it stimulates collagen and promotes elasticity.

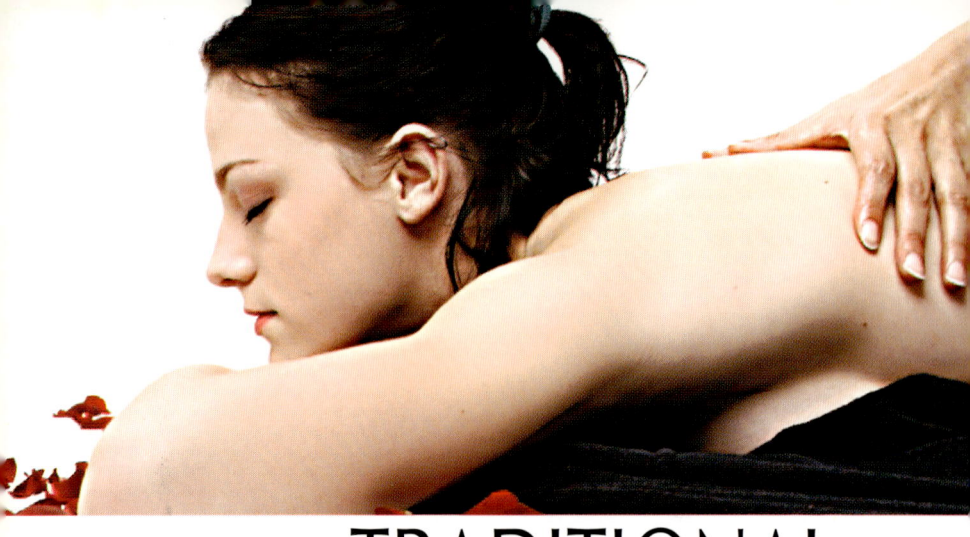

TRADITIONAL INDIAN SPA
TREATMENTS

SPAS

Almost all spas in India offer a spectrum of authentic and traditional Indian wellness treatments and experiences in a stylish and soothing ambience. The philosophy behind the treatments is the well-being of mind, body and spirit which is the key to personal fulfilment. The holistic treatments develop the mind and body to work in unison. This unique approach combines the art of ancient eastern knowledge with the best of western technologies.

India is a land where traditional rejuvenation and healing therapies have been used for centuries. Besides dealing with principles for maintaining health, Ayurveda has also developed a wide range of therapeutic measures to combat illness.

Traditional Rajasthan Ubtan

It is a ritual practised by young royal brides in preparation for their wedding day. This treatment starts with a paste made from the most natural ingredients, like turmeric, neem, etc. Mixed with milk, the exfoliation process helps to remove dead skin cells and rediscover a beautiful, soft skin. A relaxing

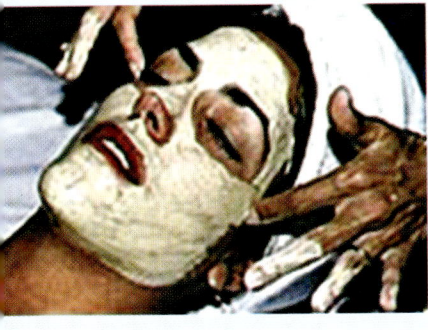

massage using sweet smelling essential oils completes this unforgettable experience.

Shirodhara

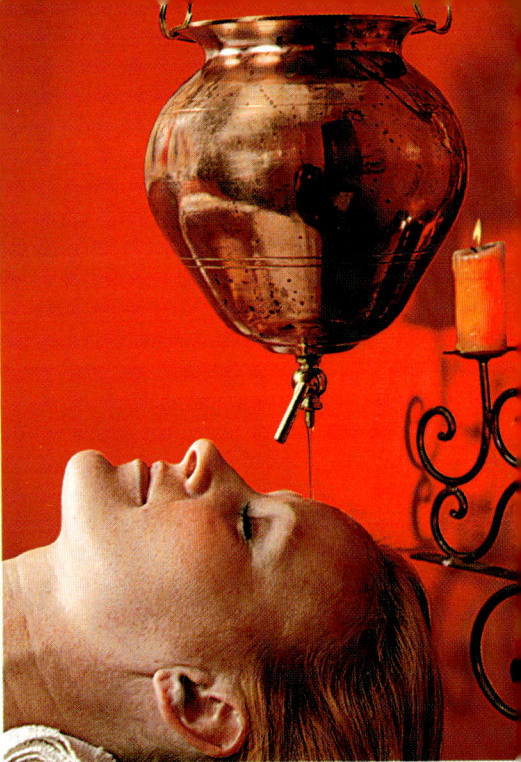

Rhythmic trickling of warm herbal oil over the forehead is believed to awaken the third eye, which in turn triggers a healing process, restoring good health. A complete sense of wellness is also induced.

Papaya Body Polish

Using mashed papaya and finely ground walnut shells, this exfoliation process will leave the skin as smooth as silk. Papaya contains enzymes such as papain, which softens and revitalises the skin when absorbed. It is an excellent choice of exfoliation to prepare the skin for better absorption of aromatherapy oils during a body massage.

Katee Vasthy

This specialised treatment relieves lower back pain due to stress and poor posture. Warm herbal oil retained in the lower back using a traditional technique followed by a back massage eases accumulated stress, and strengthens the muscles of the lower back.

Ayurvedic Massage

This traditional massage therapy uses a combination of soothing and symmetrical long strokes to regulate the circulatory and the nervous systems. The sesame-based herbal oil used in the massage heightens concentration, and leaves one feeling refreshed and rejuvenated.

Takradhara

Like Shirodhara, this therapy has a calming effect, induced by the thin, steady stream of herbal medicated buttermilk on the forehead, followed by a gentle scalp massage. This induces tranquillity, and coordinates the mind-body-soul function.

Chakra Head-Shoulder Massage

This rejuvenating massage covers the shoulder, scalp and the face, and is followed by a hot and moist fomentation. This massage concentrates on the vital energy points and provides relief to the sensory organs.

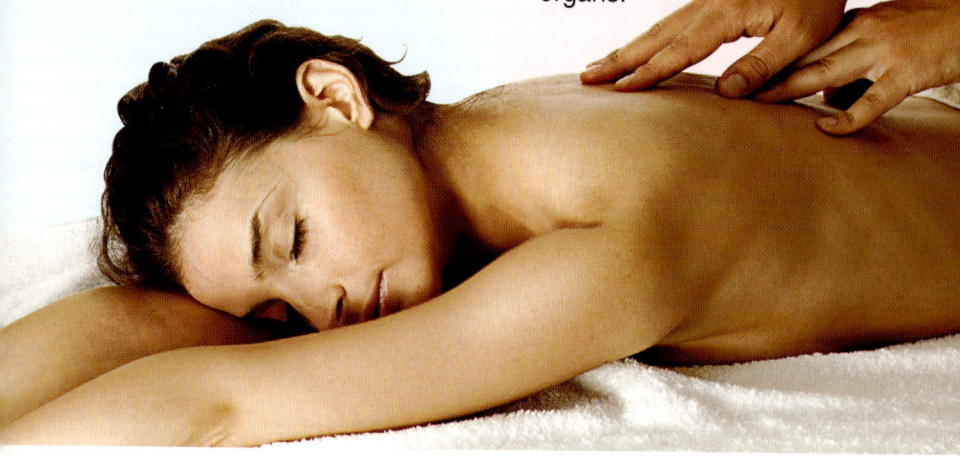

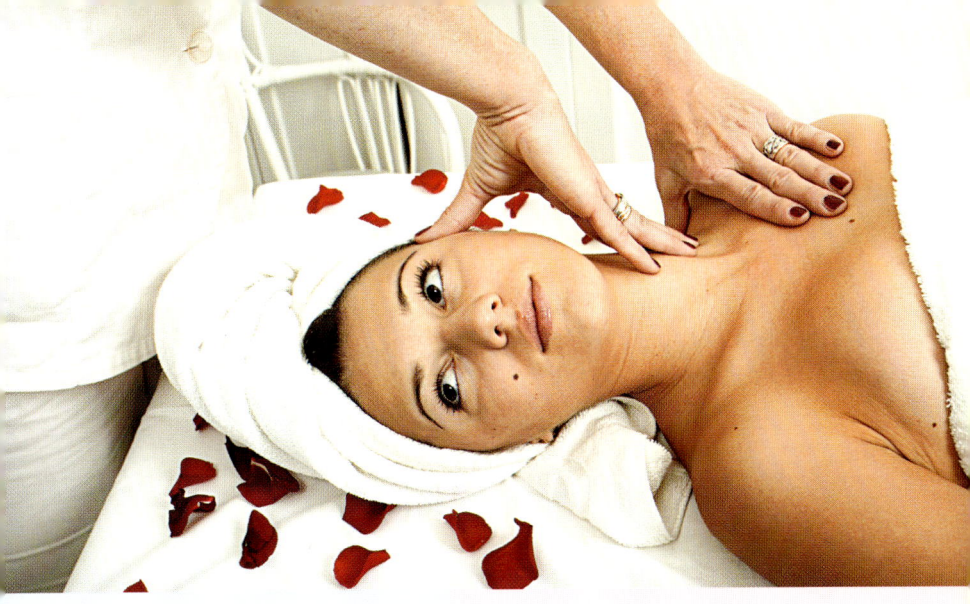

Royal Aromatic Massage

Therapists will begin this wonderful body massage, starting with a choice of essential oils. This light to medium pressure massage stimulates the lymphatic drainage system, and soothes nervous tension to bring back harmony to the body and mind. A face and scalp massage using pressure points concludes this massage to instil a sense of calm and tranquillity.

Abhyanga

This is a relaxing massage that calms the body and mind, while working impurities and toxins out of the system, using a blend of oils and herbs tailored to the individual.

Swedana

A herb-infused steam bath, Swedana removes toxins which have penetrated deep into the body's tissues.

Udvartina

Udvartina is a herbal paste used to massage, exfoliate, detoxify and condition the body.

Every spa in India has its own special spa menu that lists a number of exotic spa therapies and treatments. Besides various spa therapies, most of the spas have facilities for beauty, health, fitness, yoga, meditation, and hot and cold jacuzzis.

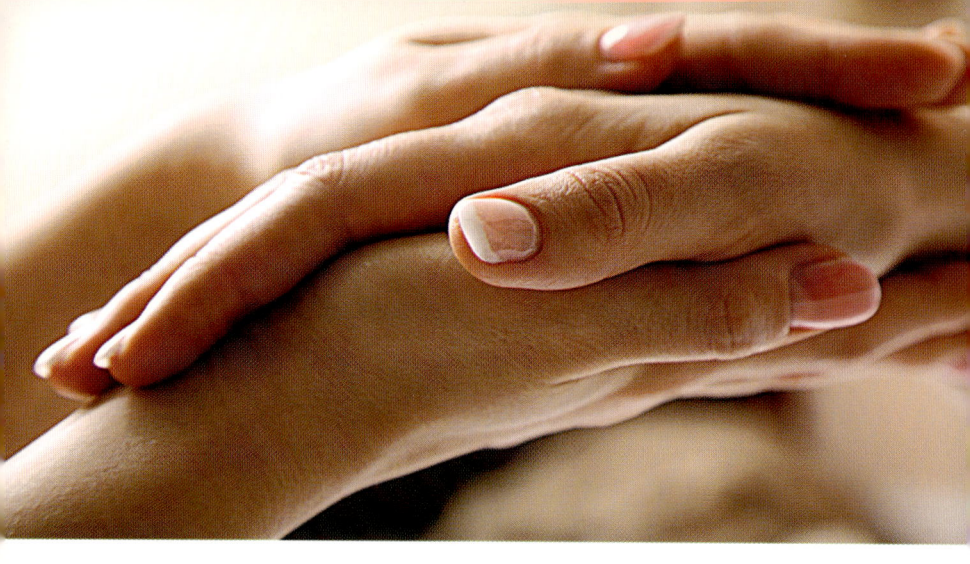

SPA MANICURE and PEDICURE

SPAS

For many women, a manicure and pedicure treatment is a luxurious treat. Having someone else take care of your nails is quick and inexpensive, but you still feel as if you are being pampered.

All spas around the world have technicians who can give you a special experience, and the secret behind well groomed hands is expert care.

The technicians in the spas focus on maintaining natural healthy nails with special attention to skin and cuticles. Spas design some unique and truly pampering hand and foot treatments that will lift the spirit and leave you feeling totally relaxed.

The Working Person's Manicure and Pedicure

This treatment is for the very busy people who have a very limited period of time. The towels are omitted here, and the massage is kept to a minimum, but when you leave, your hands and feet will look refreshed and beautiful.

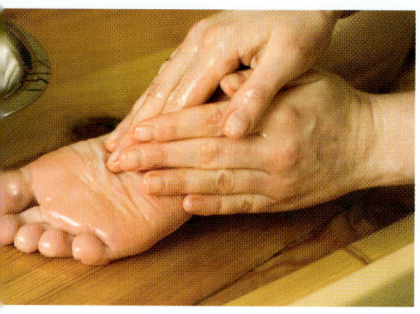

Anti-ageing Hand and Foot Treatment

This vitamin, protein and mineral-rich seaweed treatment, combined with professional hand massage, will completely hydrate, soften and nourish hands and feet. You will feel them smoother, revitalised and youthful.

☑ Cinnamon-Sugar Hand and Foot Treatment

This self-heating cinnamon-sugar scrub, that smells good enough to eat, is massaged into hands or feet while warming the body, and gently exfoliating the skin, leaving it hydrated and silky smooth.

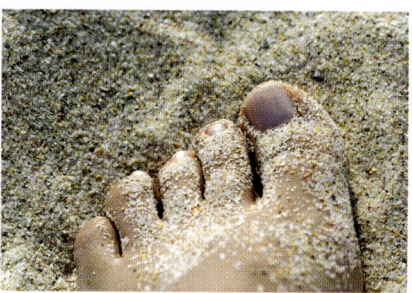

☑ Moor Mud Therapeutic Hand and Foot Treatment

This puts life back into tired hands or feet. It softens calluses, improves circulation and revitalises neglected skin. It helps to relieve pain caused by arthritis, joint and muscle pain.

Nails and Toes Ultimate Spa Treatment

Indulge in this ultimate hand and foot spa. The treatment includes a relaxing scrub, followed by a mask, then a massage. The technician tends to your hands, nails, cuticles, and then from heel to toe, using rich creams and lotions.

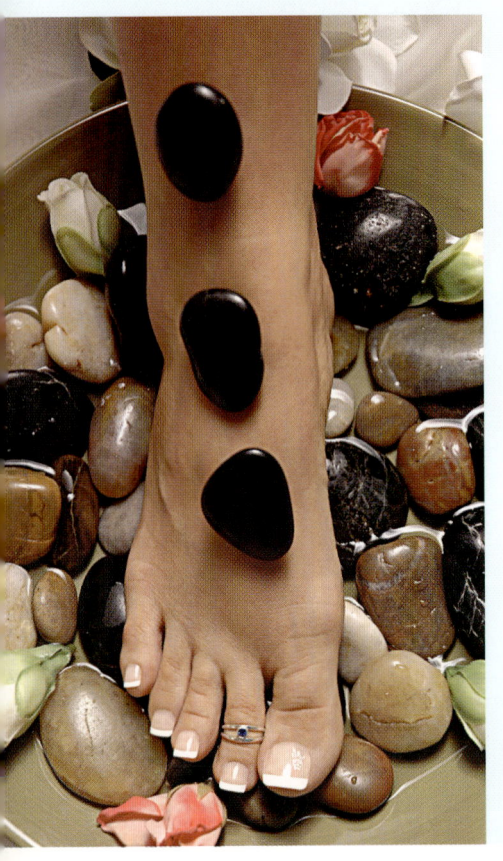

Wentworth Classic Manicure

Make a statement with well-groomed nails. The manicurist will cleanse and shape your nails, condition the cuticles, massage, and then finish off with buff or polish. Both men and women can avail of this treatment.

Deluxe Manicure

Start by selecting your preference of scent from a delightfully tantalising menu. First your hands are groomed, then exfoliated with the aroma-scented salt scrub and complementing oil. Then a warm towel wrap is applied which proves very therapeutic and hydrating.

Peppermint and Lemon Hand Luxury

Begin with a peppermint soak, followed by a peppermint and lemon exfoliation. Next, you will receive a nourishing peppermint and lemon lotion massage followed by a warm, moist towel application. Lastly, the nails are groomed and polished.

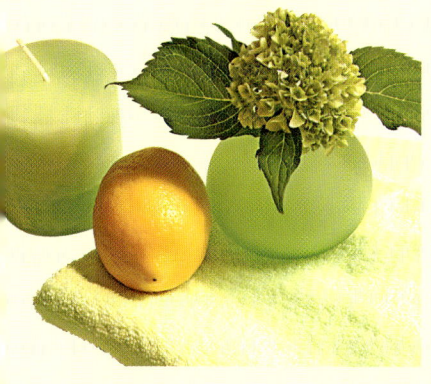

Deluxe Spa Manicure and Paraffin Duet

After choosing your fragrance from the menu, sit back, relax and enjoy a soaking, exfoliating and proper grooming, as warm oil is massaged from your hands up to your elbows. Then, your hands are dipped into warm paraffin, helping the oil to penetrate into the deep layers of your skin. Once the paraffin is peeled off from your hands, you are given a wonderfully relaxing massage.

Ultimate Spa Manicure

This manicure is a 45 minutes of pure hand-pampering delight. Your cuticles are soaked in hot oil, and then warm paraffin is poured over the hands. Then warm mitts are placed over hands for optimum hydration and softness. Also included is a loofah scrub mask to gently exfoliate the hands and arms, pure essential aromatherapy oils, a sleep-inducing hand and arm massage, and shaping of cuticles and nails. And, of course, the polish of your choice.

Golden Spa Manicure

Golden spa manicure is truly an extra special gift to yourself. Soak your hands in a floral-laced bath

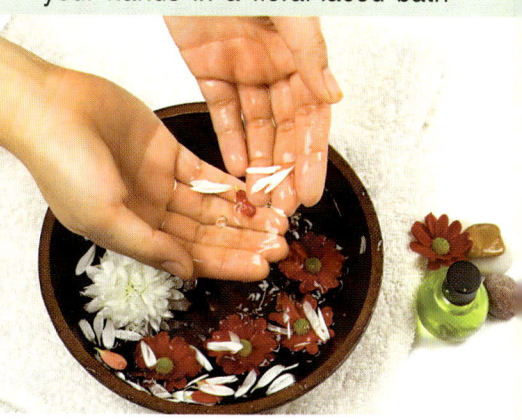

filled with fragrant oils and bath salts. Then your hands and lower arms are slathered with a mask and allowed to rest. This mask is removed with warm towels, and then your arms and hands receive a generous massage. The nails are shaped, the cuticles are groomed, and your choice of nail lacquer is applied.

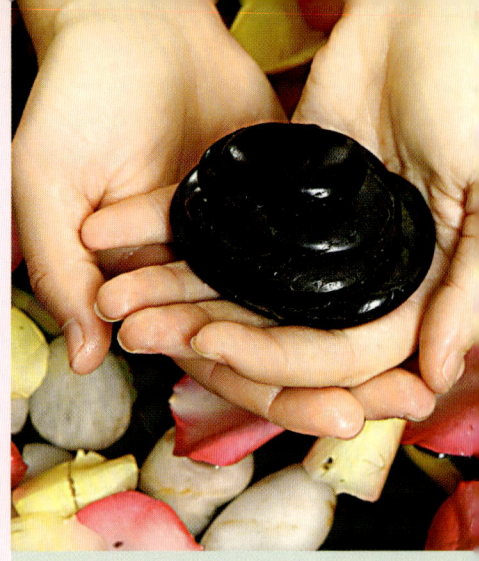

Protein Manicure

This manicure helps to nurture, heal and maintain strong, healthy nails. It includes an effervescent aroma soak, honey-almond hand exfoliation, steamy towel wraps and luxurious massage. Nails are treated with a protein solution and basecoat, and then polished to perfection.

Men's Manicure

It focuses on the cuticles and dry overworked and under-cared hands. A warm, mineral soak will allow the hands to begin the healing process. It is followed by an exfoliation, relaxing massage, and ends with a warm paraffin mask.

Hot Stone Manicure

Sit back and relax while your nails are groomed, then dipped into paraffin. Next, your hands will be massaged with hot stones up to your elbows to achieve the ultimate in relaxation. This is followed by a moisturiser, and hot towel application. At the end nails are painted to perfection.

Glycolic Manicure

This helps your hands to look more youthful and healthy. During this treatment, glycolic acid is applied on top of hands. It helps to reduce sun spots, freckles and 'brown spots' often evident as we age.

Aromatherapy Manicure

The ultimate manicure includes an exfoliation with spa sea salts, a massage with collagen-based aromatherapy cream, and a dip in hot paraffin wax, covered with mitts to create maximum absorption of nutrients.

Sea Mud Wrap Pedicure

Organic seaweed mud wrap is used to increase circulation. The treatment also includes a sea salt scrub, whirlpool footbath, biological exfoliant peel, foot care massage, paraffin and polish.

Ultimate Spa Pedicure

This is a 75-minute ped-pampering delight. Soak those precious feet in the whirlpool jet tub with essential aromatherapy oils. It includes callus-softening and removal, cuticle and nail shaping, and an almond loofah scrub and foot mask. The feet are bathed in warm paraffin, and placed in heated towel wraps for the softest, smoothest skin imaginable.

Glycolic Pedicure

This service begins with foot hydration to soften any dead or calloused skin. The pedicurist then uses a glycolic peel treatment to remove extra layers of calloused and dead skin. Moisturisers are then massaged into your feet before a finished coat of polish is applied.

Dead Sea Mud Pedicure

This ultimate spa pedicure begins with hydration, and then includes an intensive peeling with glycolic acid. Your feet are then wrapped with Dead Sea mud to remineralise, detoxify and moisturise your feet. After feet and lower leg massage, your nails are groomed for a perfect look.

Paraffin Pedicure

This is a wonderful treatment for your feet. The pedicure begins with an invigorating exfoliation with a honey-almond scrub. Your feet are dipped into warm and silky moisturising paraffin, then wrapped

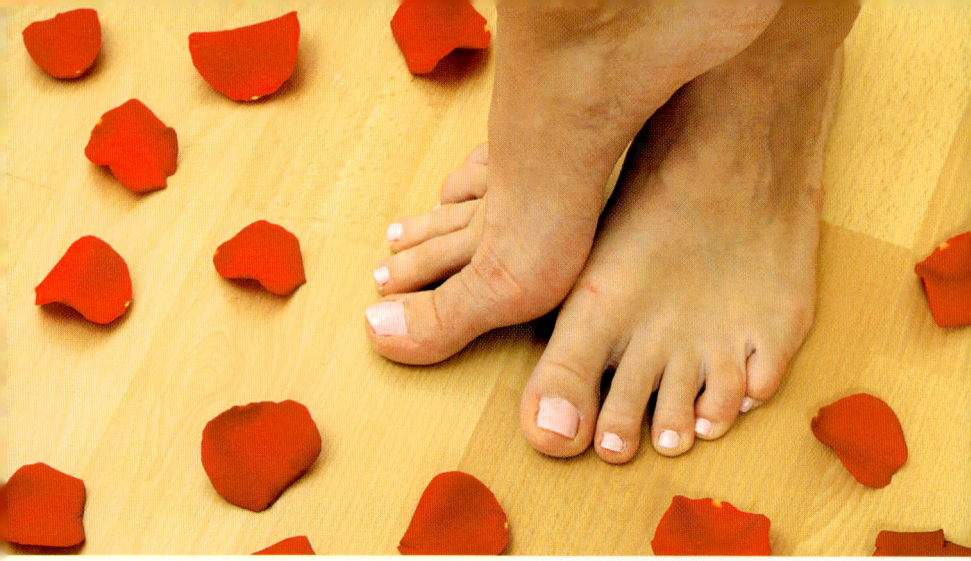

and surrounded with heat. The paraffin seals, locking in moisture, and is easily removed to reveal a soft, supple skin. This is a perfect treatment for dry, rough or chapped skin.

Aromatherapy Pedicure

This is an ultimate pedicure in which you indulge in essential aroma oils, Dead Sea salt scrub, massage with a thick collagen cream, and a dip in hot peach paraffin wax, then the feet are covered with booties for maximum absorption of nutrients.

Holistic Pedicure

This most luxurious pedicure begins with a whirlpool soak and a 30-minute foot massage using reflexology techniques to benefit all areas of the body. This therapy helps relieve stress and tension through foot pressure point massage. The technician finishes with moisturisers and a perfect pedicure.

Hawaiian Hot Ash Treatment

This comprises a full luxury pedicure using hot ash, giving your feet a wonderfully stimulating treatment that leaves you feeling as if you are walking on air with silken feet!

Feet are the most ignored area of our bodies, but they deserve better. Try a pedicure and give them an invigorating treat.

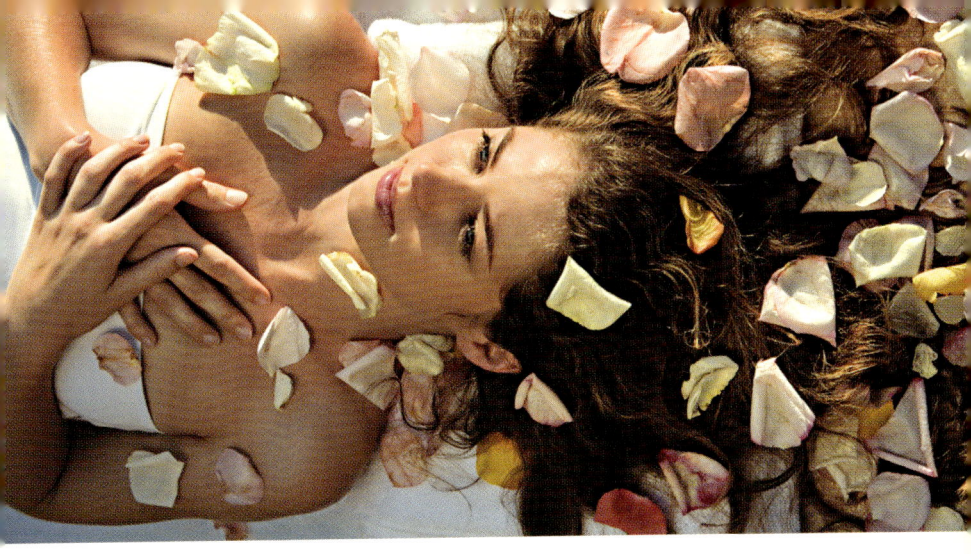

SPA HAIR and OTHER TREATMENTS

SPAS

Beauty treatments do not end with body scrubs, massages, facials, manicure or pedicure. Hair also needs equal attention and care. Spas offer you a variety of treatments that include: haircut, shampoo and conditioning, deep conditioning, blow dry, hair styling, perming, henna, colour or highlighting, straightening, crimpling, ironing, roller setting, root touch-up, scalp massage, mousse and gel application, hair setting lotion and spray application, and so on.

Hair, just like skin, are the most sensitive part of our body, and their care should never be neglected.

Hair and Scalp Treatment

This treatment is designed to renew hair to a healthy, shining state, and includes a purifying and enriching scalp renewal treatment, a neck and scalp massage, renewing shampoo and lightweight cream detangler or finishing rinse.

Special essential nutrients are scientifically formulated to enhance circulation, nourish roots, and leave the hair healthy, soft and glossy.

Scalp Analysis and Treatment

This indepth, customised treatment with a specialist includes analysis and diagnosis of your specific hair and scalp needs, a purifying and enriching scalp renewal treatment, scalp and hair oil nourishment, a relaxing neck and scalp massage, customised scalp treatment and shampoo with a nourishing conditioner, completing the treatment with a special finishing rinse, and anti-dehydrating and protective styling products. Whether you choose a 15-minute hair and scalp renewal, or full hair and scalp analysis and treatment with a specialist, the team of trained professionals will provide you with added and long-term benefits.

Scalp Oil Massage

To begin the process, a licensed cosmetologist will examine your hair and scalp. The treatment starts with a soothing scalp massage using warm oil. The oil is then left on the

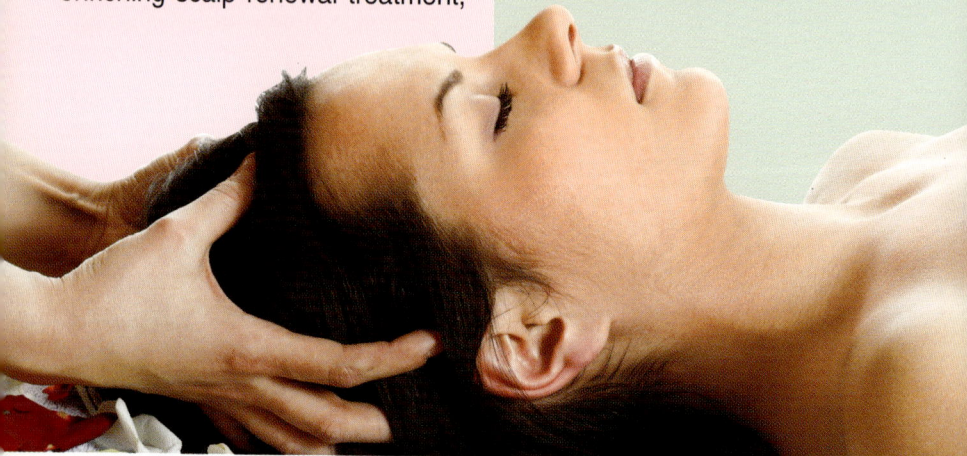

hair, and wrapped in a warm towel while you have your feet and hands attended to. This is followed by an exfoliation. A deep conditioning and balancing mask is applied, replenishing moisture to your hair and scalp.

Conditioning

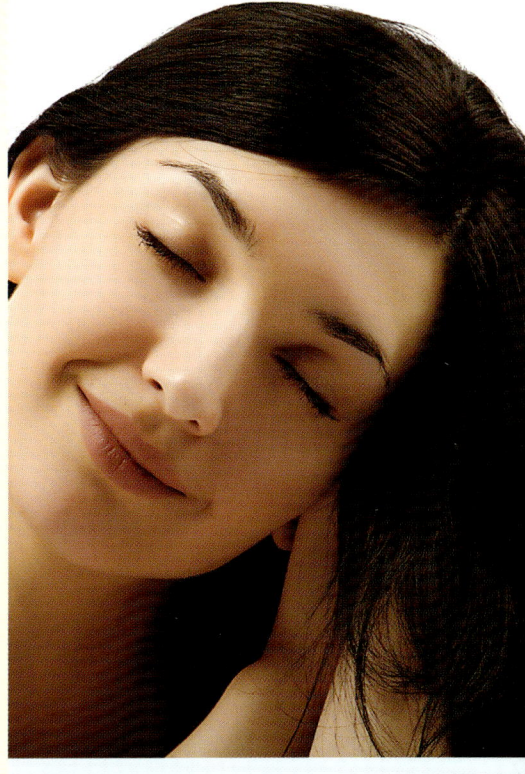

This is one of the best ways to relax. A spa hair treatment makes for a great conditioning treatment for your hair, and a relaxing day at the same time. Try it and make your stressed hair (because of hair colour, sun, wind, blow drying, etc.) silky, shiny and bouncy. Enjoy the shampooing of your hair with a cleansing shampoo.

If you have coarse, frizzy or very curly hair, have a moisturising or hydrating treatment. This is usually thick and creamy, and will help to soften your hair and improve its flexibility.

If you have permed, colour-treated or sun bleached hair, then a protein reconstruction conditioner is used.

In badly damaged hair, these treatments are given frequently to sustain the added strength. Your hair will be thoroughly coated with the conditioner while a comb is run through your hair. Then your hair is wrapped in a towel or plastic bag or cap to keep the hair and scalp warm for 10 minutes. When your hair is rinsed, you will find it stronger, silkier and shinier.

Ionic Conditioning Treatment

This is the latest in ionic hair care technology. It restores the hair's vitality and nourishes it back into a state of health after one short treatment. It leaves your hair feeling soft and silky.

☑ Rosemary-Honey-Oil Conditioner

This nourishing conditioner blends two ingredients from nature — honey for shine and olive oil for moisture — and is enhanced with the essential oil of rosemary to stimulate hair growth. It is then massaged into the scalp until it is completely and evenly distributed. It is then left to nourish and condition for half an hour which will ultimately give you shinier, softer and healthier hair the natural way.

☑ Hair Retexturising

This is a revolutionary treatment for straightening hair through the process of negative ionisation. It uses scientific technology in conjunction with a naturally active mineral shampoo to form water molecule clusters that break down into micro-fine particles allowing moisture to penetrate deep into the hair shaft. Hair is renewed, restored and rehydrated to a fine lustre and glow.

☑ Damaged Hair Treatment

This is a specially designed treatment to offer hair and scalp relief from the damaging effects of blow drying, curling instruments and improper hair care products. It includes purifying and enriching scalp renewal treatment, using rare ingredients such as phyto-vitamins, lipids, tea tree oil and rich oil extracts from exotic Himalayan seeds; a relaxing neck and scalp massage; a moisturising shampoo and conditioner; a special finishing rinse, and hydrating and protective styling products. This luxurious rejuvenation ritual restores and repairs even the most severely damaged hair.

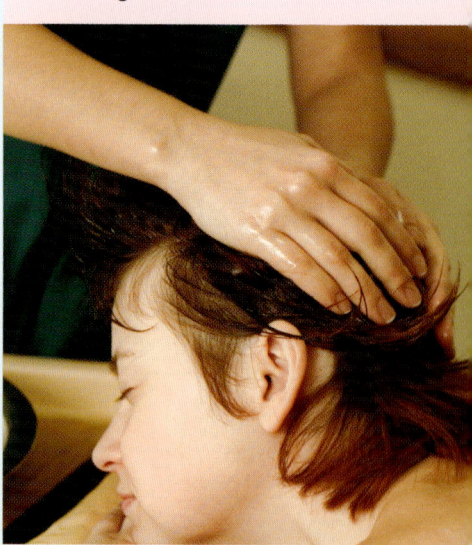

Aromatherapy Treatment

This is a deep conditioning, hot aromatherapy hair treatment. Pressure points on the neck and shoulders, as well as the entire scalp are massaged to stimulate circulation and help de-stress the body and mind. You may choose to include a shampoo, blow dry and style.

Dandruff Treatment

It requires a necessary professional treatment that corrects the problem of dandruff. This treatment consists of a purifying and enriching scalp renewal treatment, a circulatory neck and scalp massage, controlling gel treatment, a deep cleansing shampoo and lightweight cream detangler or finishing rinse.

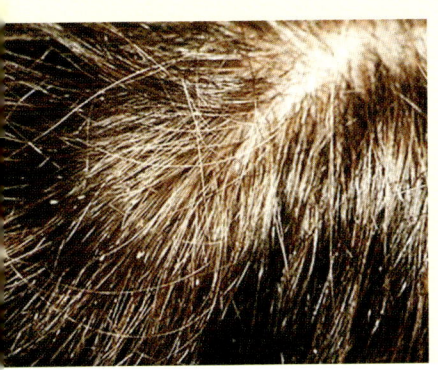

Beer Hair Rinse

Beer hair rinse consists of distilled water, apple cider vinegar, lemon essential oil, beer (even a stale one would do), rosemary essential oil and calendula essential oil. It provides protein to make your hair shiny, thicker and healthy.

Thinning Hair Treatment

Many factors in a person's life can contribute to hair thinning and loss. This particular treatment addresses the problem and provides results. The process includes a purifying and enriching scalp renewal treatment, a circulatory neck and scalp massage, treatment gel, specific treatment shampoo, finishing rinse and thinning hair treatment.

Treatment for Oily Hair

Drawing upon the naturally astringent qualities of cucumber extract with amaranth tea, this hair treatment is ideal for cleansing and removing oil and product build-up without stripping hair of its normal sheen. A rosemary mint conditioner promotes thicker and healthier hair.

Treatment for Dry or Chemically-treated Hair

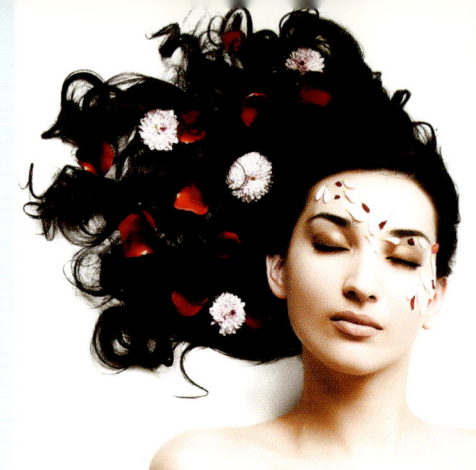

Papaya shampoo serves to moisturise and strengthen hair with the added benefit of preventing split ends. Rich in vitamins and minerals, this treatment is further reinforced with a tri-wheat reconstructor to add moisture without weighing hair down.

Another combination could be primrose and sage. A mild treatment, it helps prevent split ends, and strengthens hair cuticles through the nutrients found in primrose, chamomile and whole wheat. The sage weightless conditioner leaves your hair soft and tangle free.

Yet another treatment might be soya protein for revival of dry and chemically treated hair.

Treatment for Sensitive Scalp

A primrose and tea reliever is a good treatment for a sensitive scalp. Tree oil is beneficial to the scalp in more ways than one. Its natural anti-bacterial and anti-fungal qualities help to relieve flaking while the vitamin E found within the oil works in soothing the scalp. The addition of rosemary mint conditioner to the treatment further stimulates the scalp to promote thicker, healthier hair.

Another cleansing treatment for a dry and sensitive scalp would be of papaya and chamomile volumiser designed to moisturise and strengthen the hair while removing product build-up and preventing split ends.

Soya and mint enricher is suitable for all hair types. This wholesome hair and scalp treatment works wonders through the use of cucumber which thoroughly cleanses and strengthens the hair.

Henna Treatment

Henna is more than just a dye. The henna plant conditions and polishes hair. It prevents hair loss, combats dandruff, and provides a shiny, healthy texture to all hair types. Known for its curative as well as conditioning abilities, a specially prepared henna is used in the treatment of falling hair and dandruff.

Henna powder, amla (gooseberry) powder, egg, coffee powder, tea leaf, lemon, curd and oil are used for this herbal mixture. It removes and prevents dandruff, promotes hair growth and prevents hair loss, conditions the hair, promotes the health of the hair by keeping the scalp healthy, adds lustre to the hair, and has a cooling and soothing effect on the scalp.

Hair Removal Services

The anti-microbial method of hair removal prevents pain and redness that result from wax treatments. The use of a soya-based hair removal system is guaranteed to be gentler than wax, and excellent for a sensitive skin. This special formula not only removes unwanted hair without the redness and bumps that sometimes accompany it, but will actually leave you with softer, smoother skin.

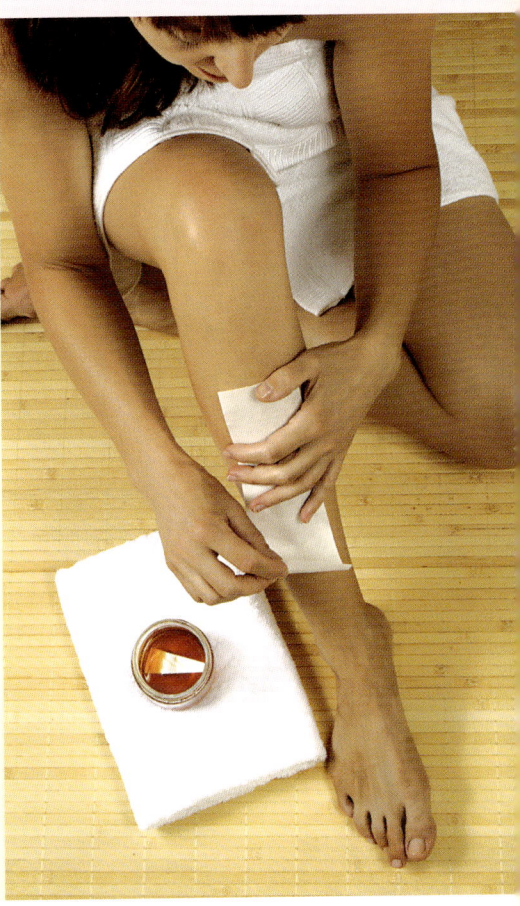

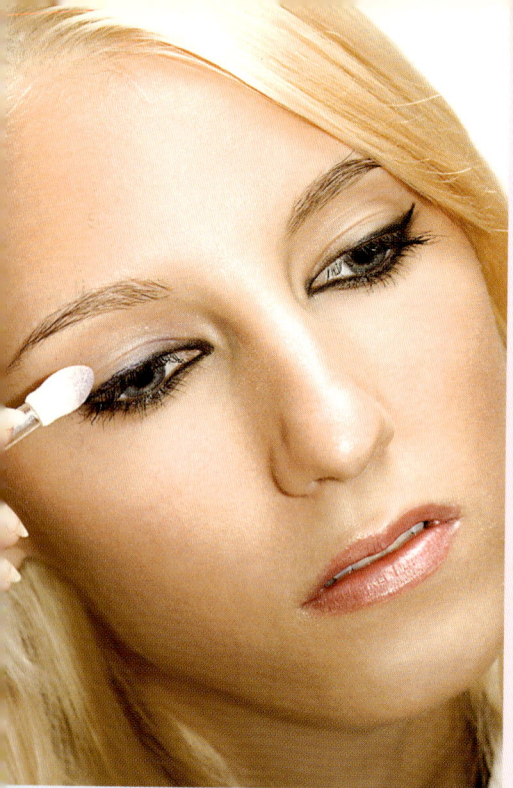

strong sensitivity. The eye area is the first to show signs of ageing. Spas offer specific treatments to help hydrate and reduce puffiness, irritation and fine lines.

The Aromatis Eye Contour treatment, a highly moisturising treatment, reduces the appearance of fine lines, wrinkles and 'crow's feet', while decongesting the eye area. It also stimulates micro circulation.

You can have your eyelashes and eyebrows tinted with combinal tint which is permanent for six to eight weeks. This defines or corrects brow shapes, and emphasises your lashes with intensified colours. Sparse eyebrows, either as a result of nature or over-tweezing, and non-existent brows caused, for example, by alopecia areata, short, uneven or irregular or ill-defined brow lines can be corrected.

Waxing

All spas provide waxing facilities for legs, arms, underarms and eyebrows.

Some other treatments to enhance your beauty are given below.

Eye Care Treatments

The eye contour area is the most delicate skin area of the face. Characterised by low blood and lymphatic circulation, this area is often dehydrated and suffers from

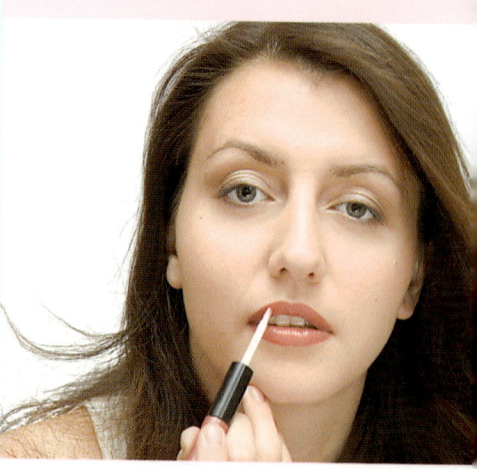

Lips

The shape of the lip can be improved, and imperfections, such as arched, flat or asymmetrical lips, can be corrected. This gentle procedure is done by hand, with no machines or injections. A topical numbing agent is applied to desensitise the area.

Semi-permanent Make-up

This type of make-up is ideal for people who live active lives, for those who are allergic to cosmetics, and those who have difficulty applying make-up, or those who wear contact lens.

Otherwise known as micro-pigmentation, this semi-permanent make-up enhances natural looks. This make-up, being carried out with needles and pigments or dyes, is sometimes marketed as permanent, creating confusion. In practical terms, it means that make-up will not be there forever, but whilst it is there, it cannot be easily erased or removed. Semi-permanent make-up will fade over time as the pigment is inserted only into the upper layer of the dermis. As the skin gets replaced over a period of two or three years, the colour fades.

Enjoy all the benefits that spas pamper you with. Relax and make the most of the rejuvenating treatments meted out there.

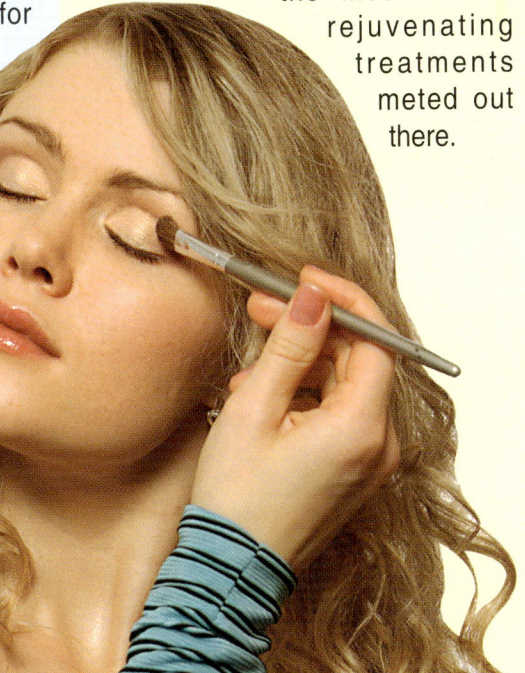